Tumors of the Ear and Lateral Skull Base: Part 2

Editors

MATTHEW L. CARLSON
GEORGE B. WANNA

OTOLARYNGOLOGIC CLINICS OF NORTH AMERICA

www.oto.theclinics.com

June 2015 • Volume 48 • Number 3

ELSEVIER

1600 John F. Kennedy Boulevard • Suite 1800 • Philadelphia, Pennsylvania, 19103-2899

http://www.oto.theclinics.com

OTOLARYNGOLOGIC CLINICS OF NORTH AMERICA Volume 48, Number 3
June 2015 ISSN 0030-6665, ISBN-13: 978-0-323-39219-8

Editor: Joanne Husovski
Developmental Editor: Susan Showalter

Otolaryngologic Clinics of North America (ISSN 0030-6665) is published bimonthly by Elsevier, Inc., 360 Park Avenue South, New York, NY 10010-1710. Months of issue are February, April, June, August, October, and December. Business and Editorial Offices: 1600 John F. Kennedy Blvd., Suite 1800, Philadelphia, PA 19103-2899. Customer Service Office: 6277 Sea Harbor Drive, Orlando, FL 32887-4800. Periodicals postage paid at New York, NY and additional mailing offices. Subscription prices is $365.00 per year (US individuals), $692.00 per year (US institutions), $175.00 per year (US student/resident), $485.00 per year (Canadian individuals), $876.00 per year (Canadian institutions), $540.00 per year (international individuals), $876.00 per year (international institutions), $270.00 per year (international & Canadian student/resident). Foreign air speed delivery is included in all *Clinics'* subscription prices. All prices are subject to change without notice. **POSTMASTER:** Send address changes to *Otolaryngologic Clinics of North America*, Elsevier Health Sciences Division, Subscription Customer Service, 3251 Riverport Lane, Maryland Heights, MO 63043. **Telephone: 1-800-654-2452 (U.S. and Canada); 314-447-8871 (outside U.S. and Canada). Fax: 314-447-8029. E-mail: journalscustomerservice-usa@elsevier.com (for print support); journalsonlinesupport-usa@elsevier.com (for online support).**

Reprints. For copies of 100 or more of articles in this publication, please contact the Commercial Reprints Department, Elsevier Inc., 360 Park Avenue South, New York, NY 10010-1710. Tel.: 212-633-3874; Fax: 212-633-3820; E-mail: reprints@elsevier.com.

Otolaryngologic Clinics of North America is also published in Spanish by McGraw-Hill Interamericana Editores S.A., P.O. Box 5-237, 06500 Mexico D.F., Mexico.

Otolaryngologic Clinics of North America is covered in *MEDLINE/PubMed (Index Medicus), Current Contents/Clinical Medicine, Excerpta Medica, BIOSIS, Science Citation Index,* and *ISI/BIOMED.*

PROGRAM OBJECTIVE

The goal of the *Otolaryngologic Clinics of North America* is to provide information on the latest trends in patient management, the newest advances; and provide a sound basis for choosing treatment options in the field of otolaryngology.

TARGET AUDIENCE

All practicing physicians and healthcare professionals who provide patient care to otolaryngologic patients.

LEARNING OBJECTIVES

Upon completion of this activity, participants will be able to:
1. Review the management of schwannomas of the ear and lateral skull base.
2. Discuss treatment of non-schwannoma tumors, such as chordomas, chondrosarcomas, and meningiomas.
3. Recognize the use for and results of stereotaxic radiosurgery as treatment for tumors of the ear and lateral skull base.

ACCREDITATION

The Elsevier Office of Continuing Medical Education (EOCME) is accredited by the Accreditation Council for Continuing Medical Education (ACCME) to provide continuing medical education for physicians.

The EOCME designates this enduring material for a maximum of 15 *AMA PRA Category 1 Credit*(s)™. Physicians should claim only the credit commensurate with the extent of their participation in the activity.

All other health care professionals requesting continuing education credit for this enduring material will be issued a certificate of participation.

DISCLOSURE OF CONFLICTS OF INTEREST

The EOCME assesses conflict of interest with its instructors, faculty, planners, and other individuals who are in a position to control the content of CME activities. All relevant conflicts of interest that are identified are thoroughly vetted by EOCME for fair balance, scientific objectivity, and patient care recommendations. EOCME is committed to providing its learners with CME activities that promote improvements or quality in healthcare and not a specific proprietary business or a commercial interest.

The planning committee, staff, authors and editors listed below have identified no financial relationships or relationships to products or devices they or their spouse/life partner have with commercial interest related to the content of this CME activity:
Derald E. Brackmann, MD; Matthew L. Carlson, MD; Colin L. Driscoll, MD; Laurence J. Eckel, MD; Anjali Fortna; David R. Friedmann, MD; Christopher D. Frisch, MD; John G. Golfinos, MD; Bartosz Grobelny, MD; Kristen Helm; Jacob B. Hunter, MD; Joanne Husovski; Jeffrey T. Jacob, MD; Jeffrey R. Janus, MD; Jack I. Lane, MD; Michael J. Link, MD; Theodore R. McRackan, MD; Brian A. Neff, MD; Bruce E. Pollock, MD; Santha Priya; Alejandro Rivas, MD; J. Thomas Roland Jr, MD; Susan Showalter; William H. Slattery, MD; Reid C. Thompson, MD; Jamie J. Van Gompel, MD; George B. Wanna, MD; Kyle D. Weaver, MD; Eric P. Wilkinson, MD.

UNAPPROVED/OFF-LABEL USE DISCLOSURE

The EOCME requires CME faculty to disclose to the participants:
1. When products or procedures being discussed are off-label, unlabelled, experimental, and/or investigational (not US Food and Drug Administration [FDA] approved); and
2. Any limitations on the information presented, such as data that are preliminary or that represent ongoing research, interim analyses, and/or unsupported opinions. Faculty may discuss information about pharmaceutical agents that is outside of FDA-approved labelling. This information is intended solely for CME and is not intended to promote off-label use of these medications. If you have any questions, contact the medical affairs department of the manufacturer for the most recent prescribing information.

TO ENROLL

To enroll in the *Otolaryngologic Clinics of North America* Continuing Medical Education program, call customer service at 1-800-654-2452 or sign up online at http://www.theclinics.com/home/cme. The CME program is available to subscribers for an additional annual fee of USD 260.

METHOD OF PARTICIPATION

In order to claim credit, participants must complete the following:

1. Complete enrolment as indicated above.
2. Read the activity.
3. Complete the CME Test and Evaluation. Participants must achieve a score of 70% on the test. All CME Tests and Evaluations must be completed online.

CME INQUIRIES/SPECIAL NEEDS

For all CME inquiries or special needs, please contact elsevierCME@elsevier.com.

Contributors

EDITORS

MATTHEW L. CARLSON, MD
Assistant Professor, Division of Otology–Neurotology and Skull Base Surgery, Department of Otolaryngology-Head and Neck Surgery, Mayo Clinic School of Medicine, Mayo Clinic, Rochester, Minnesota

GEORGE B. WANNA, MD, FACS
Associate Professor, Division of Otology–Neurotology and Skull Base Surgery, Departments of Otolaryngology-Head and Neck Surgery and Neurological Surgery, Co-Director Neurotology Fellowship Program, The Otology Group of Vanderbilt, Vanderbilt University Medical Center, Vanderbilt University, Nashville, Tennessee

AUTHORS

DERALD E. BRACKMANN, MD
Associate, House Ear Clinic, Los Angeles, California

MATTHEW L. CARLSON, MD
Assistant Professor, Division of Otology–Neurotology and Skull Base Surgery, Department of Otolaryngology-Head and Neck Surgery, Mayo Clinic School of Medicine, Mayo Clinic, Rochester, Minnesota

COLIN L.W. DRISCOLL, MD
Professor of Otolaryngology, Departments of Otolaryngology-Head and Neck Surgery and Neurologic Surgery, Mayo Clinic School of Medicine, Mayo Clinic, Rochester, Minnesota

LAURENCE J. ECKEL, MD
Assistant Professor, Department of Radiology, Mayo Clinic, Rochester, Minnesota

DAVID R. FRIEDMANN, MD
Division of Otology/Neurotology and Skull Base Surgery, Department of Otolaryngology-Head and Neck Surgery, New York University School of Medicine, New York, New York

CHRISTOPHER D. FRISCH, MD
Department of Otolaryngology-Head and Neck Surgery, Mayo Clinic, Rochester, Minnesota

JOHN G. GOLFINOS, MD
Chairman, Department of Neurosurgery, New York University School of Medicine, New York, New York

BARTOSZ GROBELNY, MD
Department of Neurosurgery, New York University School of Medicine, New York, New York

JACOB B. HUNTER, MD
Fellow, Department of Otolaryngology-Head and Neck Surgery, The Otology Group of Vanderbilt, Vanderbilt University Medical Center, Nashville, Tennessee

JEFFREY T. JACOB, MD
Skull Base Fellow, Department of Neurologic Surgery, Mayo Clinic School of Medicine, Mayo Clinic, Rochester, Minnesota

JEFFREY R. JANUS, MD
Assistant Professor, Division of Otolaryngology Head and Neck Surgery, Department of Otolaryngology, Mayo Clinic, Rochester, Minnesota

JACK I. LANE, MD
Professor, Department of Radiology, Mayo Clinic, Rochester, Minnesota

MICHAEL J. LINK, MD
Professor of Neurosurgery, Departments of Otolaryngology-Head and Neck Surgery and Neurologic Surgery, Mayo Clinic School of Medicine, Mayo Clinic, Rochester, Minnesota

THEODORE R. McRACKAN, MD
House Ear Clinic, Los Angeles, California

BRIAN A. NEFF, MD
Associate Professor, Department of Otolaryngology-Head and Neck Surgery, Mayo Clinic, Rochester, Minnesota

BRUCE E. POLLOCK, MD
Professor, Departments of Neurologic Surgery and Radiation Oncology, Mayo Clinic School of Medicine, Mayo Clinic, Rochester, Minnesota

ALEJANDRO RIVAS, MD
Vanderbilt University Medical Center, Nashville, Tennessee

J. THOMAS ROLAND Jr, MD
Professor and Mendik Foundation Chairman, Department of Otolaryngology-Head and Neck Surgery, New York University School of Medicine, New York, New York

WILLIAM H. SLATTERY, MD
House Clinic, Los Angeles, California

REID C. THOMPSON, MD
Chairman and Professor of Neurological Surgery, Department of Neurosurgery, Vanderbilt University Medical Center, Nashville, Tennessee

JAMIE J. VAN GOMPEL, MD
Assistant Professor, Departments of Neurosurgery and Otolaryngology, Mayo Clinic, Rochester, Minnesota

GEORGE B. WANNA, MD, FACS
Associate Professor, Division of Otology–Neurotology and Skull Base Surgery, Departments of Otolaryngology-Head and Neck Surgery and Neurological Surgery, Co-Director Neurotology Fellowship Program, The Otology Group Of Vanderbilt, Vanderbilt University Medical Center, Vanderbilt University, Nashville, Tennessee

KYLE D. WEAVER, MD
Assistant Professor of Neurological Surgery, Department of Neurosurgery, Vanderbilt University Medical Center, Nashville, Tennessee

ERIC P. WILKINSON, MD
House Ear Clinic, Los Angeles, California

Contents

This article gives a history of the major advances that have contributed to the current management of lateral skull base lesions. These advances include changes in surgical technique, better understanding of the natural history of these lesions, and the advent of stereotactic radiosurgery. An understanding of how treatment has evolved over time improves understanding of how the current treatment methods have been developed.

Vestibular schwannomas (VS) comprise 8% of all intracranial tumors and 90% of cerebellopontine angle and internal auditory canal neoplasms. Secondary to the widespread adoption of screening protocols for asymmetrical hearing loss and the increasing use of advanced imaging, the number of VS diagnosed each year continues to rise, while the average size has declined. Microsurgery remains the treatment of choice for large tumors, however the management of small- to medium-sized VS remains highly controversial with options including observation, radiotherapy, or microsurgery. Within this chapter, the authors provide an overview of the contemporary management of VS, reviewing important considerations and common controversies.

This article reviews the relevant anatomy, pathophysiology, clinical presentation, radiographic differential, management, outcomes, and rehabilitation of patients with intralabyrinthine schwannomas.

Neurofibromatosis type 2 (NF2) is a rare syndrome characterized by bilateral vestibular schwannomas, multiple meningiomas, cranial nerve tumors, spinal tumors, and eye abnormalities. NF2 presents unique challenges to the otologist because hearing loss may be the presenting complaint leading to the diagnosis of the disorder. Care of patients with NF2 requires knowledge of all tumors and symptoms involved with the disorder. It is recommended that patients receive care in a center with expertise in NF2. The role of the neuro-otologist in this care is determined by the specialty center.

Gamma Knife stereotactic radiosurgery (GKS) has become an important
management strategy for an increasing number of patients with skull
base tumors. For select patients with lateral skull base disorders, given
the proximity to sensitive critical structures such as the brainstem, cranial
nerves, and cochlea, this technology has emerged as a first-line treatment
to achieve the paramount goals of long-term tumor control and mainte-
nance of existing neurologic function. This article reviews the indications,
technique, and results of GKS for the treatment of vestibular schwannoma
and glomus jugulare tumors, and highlights our experience in treating
these tumors at the Mayo Clinic.

OTOLARYNGOLOGIC CLINICS
OF NORTH AMERICA

RELATED INTEREST

Imaging of the Skull Base: Anatomy and Pathology
Bruno A. Policeni and Wendy R.K. Smoker, *Authors*
in
Radiologic Clinics of North America
January 2015 (Vol. 53, Issue 1)
Head and Neck Imaging
Richard H. Wiggins and Ashok Srinivasan, *Editors*

THE CLINICS ARE AVAILABLE ONLINE!
Access your subscription at:
www.theclinics.com

Preface

Tumors of the Ear and Lateral Skull Base: Part 2

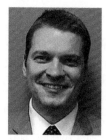 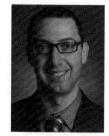

Matthew L. Carlson, MD   George B. Wanna, MD, FACS
Editors

Over the past 100 years, the evaluation and management of lateral skull base tumors have evolved tremendously. While most pathology involving the temporal bone and cerebellopontine angle is histologically benign, significant morbidity may occur as a result of disease progression or treatment. At the turn of the twentieth century, mortality from cerebellopontine angle tumor extirpation exceeded 80% and invariably resulted in substantial cranial nerve morbidity in the small percentage of those that survived the perioperative window. As a result of refinements in diagnostic imaging, microsurgical techniques, and stereotactic radiation delivery, today disease- and treatment-associated mortality approaches zero, and the majority of patients receive durable tumor control and experience minimal neurologic morbidity. Recognizing the significant advantages of multidisciplinary care, most centers utilize the collective expertise of neurotologists, neurosurgeons, and radiation oncologists in the treatment of patients with lateral skull base tumors.

It is a great honor and privilege to guest-edit this important two-part issue of *Otolaryngologic Clinics of North America* entitled, "Tumors of the Ear and Lateral Skull Base." We were extremely fortunate to assemble a cadre of world-renowned experts to share their clinical insights and knowledge regarding the complex and evolving treatment of lateral skull base disease. Part 2 is primarily dedicated to tumors of the cerebellopontine angle and petroclival region, including vestibular schwannoma, intralabyrinthine schwannoma, neurofibromatosis type 2, nonschwannoma tumors of the cerebellopontine angle, primary tumors of the facial nerve, petroclival meningioma, chondrosarcoma, and chordoma, and an overview of stereotactic radiosurgery for

Otolaryngol Clin N Am 48 (2015) xiii–xiv
http://dx.doi.org/10.1016/j.otc.2015.04.001
0030-6665/15/$ – see front matter © 2015 Published by Elsevier Inc.
oto.theclinics.com

tumors of the lateral skull base. We extend our sincerest gratitude to each contributing author for dedicating a significant amount of time and effort toward the completion of this comprehensive two-part issue.

Matthew L. Carlson, MD
Division of Otology–Neurotology & Skull Base Surgery
Mayo Clinic
Gonda Building, 12S-ENT
200 First Street
Rochester, MN 55905, USA

George B. Wanna, MD, FACS
Division of Otolaryngology-Head & Neck Surgery and Neurological Surgery
Neurotology Fellowship Program
The Otology Group of Vanderbilt
Vanderbilt University Medical Center
1215 21st Avenue South
7209 Medical Center East, South Tower
Nashville, TN 37232, USA

E-mail addresses:
carlson.matthew@mayo.edu (M.L. Carlson)
george.wanna@Vanderbilt.edu (G.B. Wanna)

Historical Perspective on Evolution in Management of Lateral Skull Base Tumors

Theodore R. McRackan, MD, Derald E. Brackmann, MD*

KEYWORDS

- Lateral skull base tumors • Lateral skull base lesions • Acoustic neuroma
- Schwannoma • Glomus jugulare • Jugular paraganglioma • Meningioma
- Stereotactic radiosurgery

KEY POINTS

- During the first 100 years of lateral skull base surgery, the mortality has decreased from 80% to the current rate of less than 0.5% through the efforts of Cushing, Dandy, House, and numerous others.
- The invention of modern imaging techniques (eg, MRI) has allowed a better understanding of the natural history of lateral skull base lesions.
- Modern deescalated radiosurgery doses of 12 to 13 Gy have maintained excellent tumor control rates (>90%) with decreased associated morbidity.
- Surgical resection has become less aggressive, favoring preserved facial nerve function rather than complete tumor resection.

INTRODUCTION

The history of lateral skull base tumor management is best understood through the history of acoustic neuroma (AN) surgery. Like most lateral skull base lesions, ANs were initially thought to be unresectable. Surgical resection of lateral skull base tumors had a tumultuous course before arriving at the extremely low mortalities seen with modern surgery. As understanding of these lesions continues to advance so does our treatment algorithm. This article describes the major turning points in the treatment of lateral skull base lesions and how treatment strategies continue to evolve.

EARLY HISTORY OF ACOUSTIC NEUROMA SURGERY

ANs were among the first lesions to be anatomically localized based on symptomatology alone. ANs therefore played a major role in neurosurgical history. The earliest

Disclosures: None.
House Ear Clinic, 2100 West 3rd Street, Los Angeles, CA 90057, USA
* Corresponding author. House Ear Clinic, 2100 West 3rd Street, Suite 111, Los Angeles, CA 90057.
E-mail address: dbrackmann@houseclinic.com

Otolaryngol Clin N Am 48 (2015) 397–405
http://dx.doi.org/10.1016/j.otc.2015.02.002
0030-6665/15/$ – see front matter © 2015 Elsevier Inc. All rights reserved.

Abbreviations

AN   Acoustic neuroma
GK   Gamma Knife
WRS   Word recognition scores

descriptions of cerebellopontine angle lesions causing deafness and facial numbness date back to the mid–nineteenth century.[1,2] However, it was not until the later part of that century that the first attempts at AN resection were made.

The first reported surgical attempt was by Charles McBurney in 1891, who opened a suboccipital plate with a mallet and chisel.[3] Because of excessive cerebellar swelling, no tumor could be removed and the patient died 12 days later. Soon thereafter (1894), an account from Charles Ballance described the first successful complete removal of an AN.[4] Exposure was performed through a suboccipital approach and tumor was removed using blunt finger dissection. During this earliest era of AN surgery, the surgical mortality approached 80%, with high operative morbidity affecting the few patients who survived.[5] It is clear that if posterior fossa surgery were to continue, significant advances would be needed.

More modern surgical techniques were ushered in during the Harvey Cushing era (early 1900s). His technique included using an extended bilateral suboccipital approach and a belief that only the core of the tumor could be safely resected.[6] He postulated that, by leaving the tumor capsule intact, cranial nerve function would be preserved and the brainstem vasculature would be left undisturbed. Cushing also advocated for the use of delicate and meticulous surgical technique, decreased cerebellar retraction, and the importance of relieving cerebrospinal fluid pressure to improve operative space. Along with the use of bone wax and electrocautery for hemostasis, this allowed him to decrease the surgical mortality to 20% in his lifetime.[6–8]

Although there was significant overlap with Cushing, the Walter Dandy era saw the increased use of diagnostic imaging to guide surgical technique. In 1918, Dandy invented ventriculography, which allowed neurosurgeons to identify the approximate location and size of brain tumors for the first time.[6,9] This ability was further advanced 1 year later by his development of pneumoencephalography.[6] In addition, Dandy, developed the more modern unilateral suboccipital approach using a smaller bone flap. He also created a schism between himself and Cushing by advocating and successfully performing total tumor excision.[10,11] Improving on Cushing's advances, Dandy was able to advance the modern surgical era.

The introduction of the operative microscope by William House[12] in 1961 changed neurosurgery forever. This microscope allowed improved viewing of the cranial nerves and blood vessels, permitting more complete tumor resection with decreased morbidity. It made facial nerve preservation with tumor resection possible for the first time. This improved vision paved the way for House to fully develop the translabyrinthine approach; unknown to House, this had been described by Panse[13] (1904) and Quix[14] (1911) decades earlier.[15] The microscope also allowed the development of the transcochlear approach as well as hearing preservation surgery in the form of the middle cranial fossa and the modern retrosigmoid approach.

Before William House's era, there was no cooperation between otologists and neurosurgeons in posterior fossa surgery. They were often vehemently opposed to their counterparts performing these surgeries. This lack of cooperation changed when William House invited William Hitselberger to join forces in treating posterior fossa lesions. The two spent countless hours together in the temporal bone laboratory cross-training to gain from each other's expertise. Over time, they created the modern collaborative neurosurgeon/neuro-otologist relationship that is now used across the world. It is easy to take this working relationship for granted in the modern era, but it is important to remember that it arose from the hard work and dedication of these two men.

The surgical treatment of meningiomas, glomus tumors, facial nerve schwannomas, petrous apex lesions, and other lateral skull base lesions was also similarly affected by the surgical advances discussed earlier. The modernization and adaptation of these surgical approaches, along with use of the operative microscope, allowed surgeons to surgically address these lesions with improved outcomes.

IMAGING

Without radiological advances, our current understanding of the size and growth characteristics of lateral skull base lesions would be deficient. It became possible to identify moderate-sized tumors with the use of positive contrast cisternography.[16] Later, the development of the Polytome Pantopaque technique allowed the diagnosis of smaller lesions confined to the internal auditory canal.[6] Although all these advances were helpful at their time, the widespread use of computer tomography and eventually MRI in the 1980s greatly improved the characterization of these lesions and ultimately became the primary diagnostic imaging study.[17] The improved identification of AN, along with improved MRI resolution, allowed physicians to better understand the natural history of skull base lesions and intervene at an earlier stage than was previously possible.

NATURAL HISTORY OF SKULL BASE LESIONS

Perhaps the greatest breakthrough in the management of lateral skull base tumors has been a better understanding of the natural growth rates of these lesions. Before this, nearly all lesions were surgically resected on diagnosis regardless of symptoms. It is now known that meningiomas, facial nerve schwannomas, and glomus tumors follow similar slow growth patterns to AN.

Multiple studies have reported the overall growth rates of ANs to vary widely, between 6% and 73%.[18] However, when data have been collected in meta-analyses, 51% of ANs show no growth, 43% to 54% grow, and 4% to 8% regress in size.[19–21]

Data from the Denmark Prospective Observational Study show that 17% of intrameatal and 28.9% of extrameatal ANs showed growth ($P<.001$). There was also a clear predilection toward growth in the first years of observation. Of those tumors that grew, most (62%–64%) grew during the first year, 23% to 28.9% grew during the second year, 5% to 10% grew during the third, and 0% to 2% grew during the fourth year of observation. When quantified, the mean growth rate for all tumors is 1 to 2 mm/y. For only those tumors that grow, this rate increases to 2 to 4 mm/y.[18] When analyzing these data, it is important to realize that there is significant selection bias. Only those tumors that could be observed without intervention were included. Therefore, any tumor that was deemed too large or symptomatic for observation (and presumptively had grown before time of presentation) was not included in the study. Therefore, the true AN growth rate may be higher than reported.

However, an improved understanding of the natural history of AN has greatly altered the treatment paradigm. Surgery was no longer the only option because a watch-and-wait approach was seen to be safe and advisable in a select group of patients. This same concept was eventually applied to other lateral skull base lesions with slow growth patterns.

RADIOTHERAPY

The next major advancement in treatment of lateral skull base lesions was the invention of stereotactic radiosurgery by Dr Lars Leksell. The first Gamma Knife (GK) unit was installed in Stockholm, Sweden, in 1968 and the first in the United States was at the University of Pittsburgh in 1987. With the publication of their seminal *New England Journal of Medicine* article, Kondziolka and colleagues[22] showed GK to be a viable treatment option for ANs. Although initial control rates were excellent, the tumor margin radiation doses ranged from 14 to 20 Gy. With these large treatment doses, there was significant associated morbidity. Some degree of facial nerve neuropathy was seen in 21% of patients and 27% developed trigeminal nerve symptoms that were statistically associated with higher doses of radiation (*P*<.003).

However, over time, the marginal tumor doses have be deescalated to 12 to 13 Gy with consistent tumor control rates greater than 90%.[23–25] Compared with studies with larger radiation doses, it seems that there is a trend toward decreased tumor shrinkage but persistent tumor stability.[22] In contrast, there has also been a dramatic decrease in the frequency of cranial neuropathy.[26–30]

Understanding of hearing loss after radiosurgery continues to evolve. For years the literature was troubled by inconsistent methods of measuring hearing preservation in addition to inadequate follow-up periods. It was initially thought that hearing loss stabilized 2 to 3 years after treatment. Numerous early studies showed that after this time period the functional hearing can be preserved in 50% to 100% of patients.[31] It is now apparent that those with serviceable hearing before treatment continue to show deterioration over time. Recent studies have shown that serviceable hearing preservation rates 8 to 10 years after treatment are 23% to 34%.[27,32]

Stereotactic radiosurgery has now been used to treat numerous lateral skull base lesions. However, perhaps the greatest impact has been on glomus jugulare tumors. Stereotactic radiosurgery has become the first line of treatment at many centers for growing symptomatic tumors because of decreased morbidity compared with surgery and comparable control rates.[33]

As understanding of the long-term outcomes of stereotactic radiosurgery become more complete, the treatment algorithm may continue to change. Radiosurgery is indicated in a select group of patient and has shown excellent control rates. However, the risks and expected outcomes should be fully understood by the recommending physician and patient before treatment.

SURGERY

With application of radiosurgery and a better understanding of the natural history of lateral skull base lesions, the indications for surgery have greatly changed over time. Before this, nearly any lesion of the lateral skull base was resected on diagnosis. Since the 1960s, the 3 main approaches to the lateral skull base (middle fossa, retrosigmoid, and translabyrinthine approach) have increasingly been refined. The creation of accurate and real-time cranial nerve monitoring, specifically facial nerve and auditory brainstem response, have improved safety and surgical proficiency. In addition, continued advances in microscope technology have improved microscopic vision, and enhanced instrumentation such as the laser and ultrasonic aspirators have greatly aided tumor resection. Collectively, these improvements have resulted in a reduction in overall mortality to 0.5%.[34]

As technology and surgical technique have improved, there has been an increased emphasis on functional preservation rather than complete resection. It has been clearly reported that postoperative facial nerve function is likely to be worse with large tumors.[35-39] This finding has led many institutions, including our own, to prefer near-total or subtotal resections to complete resection with facial nerve injury.

In our institution's data for patients with ANs greater than 2.5 cm, there is a clear trend for patients to have worse facial nerve function when receiving gross total resection.[40] Comparing facial nerve outcomes in those undergoing a near total resection, subtotal resection, and gross total resection, the percentage of those having House-Brackmann grades I and II were 97%, 96%, and 77% respectively ($P<.001$). Patients undergoing near-total resections and subtotal resections had higher rates of tumor regrowth than gross total resection but both groups had a low need for further treatment (2% and 10% vs 0%; $P<.001$). Although some clinicians advocate planned stereotactic radiation for incompletely resected large tumors, we do not.[41-45] Given the low need for retreatment seen earlier, it is our belief that, when a true subtotal or near-total resection is performed, the decreased vascularity of the tumor results in a low likelihood of tumor growth.

Similar less aggressive surgical approaches have been applied to other lateral skull base lesions. For example, surgery for facial nerve schwannomas is currently limited to decompression when patients have good facial nerve function and resection with nerve grafting when facial nerve function is poor.[46] This approach is used because of poor facial nerve outcomes when partial resections are performed. Glomus jugulare tumors have had a similar treatment progression. Rather than risk significant lower cranial nerve morbidity, surgical resection is limited to preservation of the lower cranial nerves when normal function exists. Observation versus postoperative stereotactic radiation is often used after surgery in these cases to minimize lower cranial nerve injury.

OBSERVATION

The final treatment option for any benign lateral skull base lesion is observation. With increased knowledge of the natural history of these tumors, this has become a more accepted strategy. In assessing 114 patients with ANs who we elected to receive conservative observation at our institution, 38% ultimately showed tumor growth. Most of these patients (69%) did not require intervention and were able to be followed for many years. As seen, we now take a much more conservative approach to surgery.[47]

Within the international skull base community there is an overall trend toward increased observation of lateral skull base lesions. In the report by Tan and colleagues[48] from Johns Hopkins, between 1997 and 2007 there was an increasing percentage of patients undergoing observation (10.5%–28.9%) and radiosurgery (0%–4.0%) with a decrease in operative cases (89.5%–68.0%). Similar but more dramatic trends have been seen in the United Kingdom. In the data from 2001 to 2011, the number of patients undergoing observation and radiation increased from 41% to 69% and 8% to 12%, respectively, whereas the percentage of patients having surgery decreased from 51% to 19%.[49]

Although there are well-defined data showing an increased trend toward observing ANs, similar trends have occurred with other lateral skull base lesions. As mentioned earlier, observation of other lateral skull base lesions (especially facial nerve schwannomas and glomus tumors) has increased in recent times. Like ANs, this is because of a better understanding of the natural history of these lesions and the morbidity associated with surgery.

INCIDENTAL ASYMPTOMATIC TUMORS

As the use of MRI increases and the quality of imaging improves, there has been an increased incidence of lateral skull base lesions diagnosed. Data from Denmark's national database shows that the incidence of ANs has increased from 3.1 per million in 1976 to 19.4 per million in 2008. During this time period the size at diagnosis also decreased from 30 mm to 10 mm with significantly better hearing at the time of diagnosis.[50] The increased use of imaging has led to a growing number of asymptomatic patients being incidentally diagnosed with lateral skull base lesions.

Determining the optimal treatment of this patient population can be difficult and is predicated on further testing. The first decision to be made is whether or not to intervene. The 3 main factors that guide the treatment decision are tumor size, results of audiologic testing, and age. As discussed earlier, the reported frequency of AN growth varies greatly,[18] but the rate in collected data seems to be approximately 50%.[19–21] Therefore, most of these patients should initially be observed with serial imaging.

The size of the tumor at diagnosis likely plays a significant role in determining future growth. Multiple studies have shown that tumors larger than 2 cm have a higher likelihood of future growth and may require intervention.[18,51–55] With regard to hearing, any asymptomatic patient likely has American Academy of Otolaryngology – Head and Neck Surgery class A hearing. In Denmark's data, of those patients with class A hearing at presentation, 51% maintained class A hearing and 80.8% maintained serviceable hearing over a mean follow-up of 5 years.[56] However, word recognition scores (WRS) may be more predictive of hearing outcome. With 10-year follow-up, only 31% of patients with 100% WRS at diagnosis developed WRS of less than 70%. This finding varies greatly from patients with even 90% to 99% WRS, nearly 50% of whom developed WRS of less than 70%. This decrease in WRS can occur irrespective of tumor growth.[56]

The last and most important factor is the age of the patient. Except for exceedingly rare very large tumors in asymptomatic patients, almost all tumors diagnosed in the elderly can be observed. In younger patients, this decision is more difficult and the data discussed earlier on tumor size and hearing are helpful. The presence or absence of fundal fluid along with a superior versus inferior vestibular nerve tumor can predict the success of hearing preservation surgery. Those patients with superior vestibular nerve tumors and fundal fluid on preoperative MRI are most likely to preserve hearing after surgery.[57] This information can help guide the treatment discussion with the patient and determine the best management of an individual's tumor.

Data for other lateral skull base lesions are sparse, but have are consistent with the treatment of asymptomatic ANs, especially for facial nerve schwannomas and glomus jugulare tumors, foe which surgical resection can result in significant morbidity in a previously asymptomatic patient. In these lesions, serial imaging and counseling is often the best treatment.

SUMMARY AND CURRENT TREATMENT STRATEGY

Given the changes in AN treatment over time, it is appropriate to end this article with our current treatment algorithm for ANs. We currently use the middle cranial fossa approach for younger (<65 years old) patients with tumors less than 1.5 cm and good hearing. When a patient of any age has a small tumor with poor hearing, we recommend observation. If the tumor ultimately shows growth, we recommend translabyrinthine removal in young patients and radiosurgery in the elderly. For younger patients with tumors too large for middle fossa resection but smaller than 2.5 cm with good hearing, we recommend the retrosigmoid approach; we recommend radiosurgery for the same tumor in an elderly patient with good hearing. Note that we think that radiosurgery should only be performed on tumors that have shown clear growth. In addition, regardless of hearing and age, with any tumor 3 cm or larger we recommend a translabyrinthine approach.

REFERENCES

1. Stevens GT. A case of tumor of the auditory nerve occupying the fossa of the cerebellum. Arch Otolaryngol 1879;7:171–6.
2. Toynbee J. Neuroma of the auditory nerve. Trans Path Soc London 1853;4: 259–60.
3. McBurney C, Starr MA. A contribution to cerebral surgery: diagnosis, localization and operation for removal of three tumors of the brain: with some comments upon the surgical treatment of brain tumors. Am J Med Sci 1893;55:361–87.
4. House W, House W. Historical review and problem of acoustic neuroma. Arch Otol 1964;80:601–4.
5. Van Eiselsberg A. Uber die chirurgische Behandlung der Hirntumoren. Trans Intl Cong Med 1913;7:209–17.
6. Machinis TG, Fountas KN, Dimopoulos V, et al. History of acoustic neurinoma surgery. Neurosurg Focus 2005;18(4):1–4.
7. Cushing H. The acoustic tumors. In: Intracranial tumors. Springfield (IL): Charles C Thomas; 1932. p. 85–92.
8. Cushing H. Tumors of the nervus acousticus and the syndrome of the cerebellopontine angle. Philadelphia: WB Saunders; 1917.
9. Dandy WE. Ventriculography following injection of air into the cerebral ventricles. Ann Surg 1918;68:5.
10. Dandy WE. Results of removal of acoustic tumors by the unilateral approach. AMA Arch Surg 1941;42:1026–33.
11. Dirks DD. Acoustic neuromas. In: Youmans JR, editor. Neurological surgery, vol. 5. Philadelphia: WB Saunders; 1982. p. 2967–3003.
12. House WF. Surgical exposure of the internal auditory canal and its contents through the middle, cranial fossa. Laryngoscope 1961;71:1363–85.
13. Panse R. Klinische und pathologische Mitteilungen. Arch F Ohrenh 1904;61: 251–5.
14. Quix FH. Ein Fall von translabyrintharisch operiertem tumor acusticus. Verh dt Otol Ges 1912;21:245–55.
15. Hitselberger WE, House WF. Surgical approaches to acoustic tumors. Arch Otolaryngol 1966;84:286–91.
16. Creed L, Seeger JF. Radiologic evaluation of the acoustic neuroma. Ariz Med 1984;41:739–43.
17. Wayman J, Dutcher P, Manzione J, et al. Gadolinium-DTPA-enhanced magnetic resonance scanning in cerebellopontine angle tumors. Laryngoscope 1989;99: 1167–70.
18. Nikolopoulos TP, Fortnum H, O'Donoghue G, et al. Acoustic neuroma growth: a systematic review of the evidence. Otol Neurotol 2010;31:478–85.
19. Smouha EE, Yoo M, Mohr K, et al. Conservative management of acoustic neuroma: a meta-analysis and proposed treatment algorithm. Laryngoscope 2005; 115:450–4.
20. Yamakami I, Uchino Y, Kobayashi E, et al. Conservative management, gammaknife radiosurgery, and microsurgery for acoustic neurinomas: a systematic review of outcome and risk of three therapeutic options. Neurol Res 2003;25: 682–90.
21. Selesnick SH, Johnson G. Radiologic surveillance of acoustic neuromas. Am J Otol 1998;19:846–9.
22. Kondziolka D, Lunsford LD, McLaughlin MR, et al. Long-term outcomes after radiosurgery for acoustic neuromas. N Engl J Med 1998;339:1426–33.

23. Chopra R, Kondziolka D, Niranjan A, et al. Long-term follow-up of acoustic schwannoma radiosurgery with marginal tumor doses of 12 to 13 Gy. Int J Radiat Oncol Biol Phys 2007;68:845–51.
24. Combs SE, Volk S, Schulz-Ertner D, et al. Management of acoustic neuromas with fractionated stereotactic radiotherapy (FSRT): long-term results in 106 patients treated in a single institution. Int J Radiat Oncol Biol Phys 2005;63:75–81.
25. Hasegawa T, Fujitani S, Katsumata S, et al. Stereotactic radiosurgery for vestibular schwannomas: analysis of 317 patients followed more than 5 years. Neurosurgery 2005;57:257–65.
26. Tamura M, Carron R, Yomo S, et al. Hearing preservation after gamma knife radiosurgery for vestibular schwannomas presenting with high-level hearing. Neurosurgery 2009;64(2):289–96.
27. Hasegawa T, Kida Y, Kato T, et al. Long-term safety and efficacy of stereotactic radiosurgery for vestibular schwannomas: evaluation of 440 patients more than 10 years after treatment with Gamma Knife surgery. J Neurosurg 2013;118: 557–65.
28. Kano H, Kondziolka D, Flickinger J, et al. Predictors of hearing preservation after stereotactic radiosurgery for acoustic neuromas. J Neurosurg 2009;111:863–73.
29. Massager N, Nissim O, Delbrouck C, et al. Irradiation of cochleae structures during vestibular schwannoma radiosurgery and associated hearing outcome. J Neurosurg 2007;107:733–9.
30. Yang I, Sughrue ME, Seunggu J, et al. Facial nerve preservation after vestibular schwannoma Gamma Knife radiosurgery. J Neurooncol 2009;93:41–8.
31. Yang I, Sughrue ME, Han SJ, et al. A comprehensive analysis of hearing preservation after radiosurgery for vestibular schwannoma. J Neurosurg 2010;112:851–9.
32. Carlson ML, Jacob JT, Pollock BE, et al. Long-term hearing outcomes following stereotactic radiosurgery for vestibular schwannoma: patterns of hearing loss and variables influencing audiometric decline. J Neurosurg 2013;118:579–87.
33. Guss ZD, Batra S, Limb CJ, et al. Radiosurgery of glomus jugulare tumors: a meta-analysis. Int J Radiat Oncol Biol Phys 2011;81(4):497–502.
34. McClelland S 3rd, Guo H, Okuyemi KS. Morbidity and mortality following acoustic neuroma excision in the United States: analysis of racial disparities during a decade in the radiosurgery era. Neuro Oncol 2011;13:1252–9.
35. Chen L, Chen L, Liu L, et al. Vestibular schwannoma microsurgery with special reference to facial nerve preservation. Clin Neurol Neurosurg 2009;111:47–53.
36. Falcioni M, Fois P, Taibah A, et al. Facial nerve function after vestibular schwannoma surgery. J Neurosurg 2012;115:820–6.
37. Samii M, Gerganov VM, Samii A. Functional outcome after complete surgical removal of giant vestibular schwannomas. J Neurosurg 2010;112:860–7.
38. Brackmann DE, Cullen RD, Fisher LM. Facial nerve function after translabyrinthine vestibular schwannoma surgery. Otolaryngol Head Neck Surg 2007;136: 773–7.
39. Bloch O, Sughrue ME, Kaur R, et al. Factors associated with preservation of facial nerve function after surgical resection of vestibular schwannoma. J Neurooncol 2011;102:281–6.
40. Schwartz MS, Kari E, Strickland BM, et al. Evaluation of the increased use of partial resection of large vestibular schwannomas: facial nerve outcomes and recurrence/regrowth rates. Otol Neurotol 2013;34:1456–64.
41. Fuentes S, Arkha Y, Pech-Gourg G, et al. Management of large vestibular schwannomas by combined surgical resection and gamma knife radiosurgery. Prog Neurol Surg 2008;21:79–82.

42. Iwai Y, Yamanaka K, Ishiguro T. Surgery combined with radiosurgery of large acoustic neuromas. Surg Neurol 2003;59:283–9.
43. Park CK, Jung HW, Kim JE, et al. Therapeutic strategy for large vestibular schwannomas. J Neurooncol 2006;77:167–71.
44. van de Langenberg R, Hanssens PE, van Overbeeke JJ, et al. Management of large vestibular schwannoma. Part I. Planned subtotal resection followed by Gamma Knife surgery: radiological and clinical aspects. J Neurosurg 2011; 115:875–84.
45. Yang SY, Kim DG, Chung HT, et al. Evaluation of tumour response after gamma knife radiosurgery for residual vestibular schwannomas based on MRI morphological features. J Neurol Neurosurg Psychiatry 2008;79:431–6.
46. Wilkinson EP, Hoa M, Slattery WH, et al. Evolution in the management of facial nerve schwannoma. Laryngoscope 2011;121:2065–74.
47. Fayad JN, Semaan MT, Lin J, et al. Conservative management of vestibular schwannoma: expectations based on the length of the observation period. Otol Neurotol 2014;35(7):1258–65.
48. Tan M, Myrie OA, Lin FR, et al. Trends in the management of vestibular schwannomas at Johns Hopkins 1997–2007. Laryngoscope 2009;120:144–9.
49. MacKeith SA, Kerr RS, Milford CA. Trends in acoustic neuroma management: a 20-year review of the Oxford Skull Base Clinic. J Neurol Surg B Skull Base 2013;74:194–200.
50. Standerup SE, Mirko T, Thomsen J, et al. True incidence of vestibular schwannoma? Neurosurgery 2010;67:1335–40.
51. Agrawal Y, Clark JH, Limb CJ, et al. Predictors of vestibular schwannoma growth and clinical implications. Otol Neurotol 2010;31:807–12.
52. Fucci MJ, Buchman CA, Brackmann DE, et al. Acoustic tumor growth: implications for treatment choices. Am J Otol 1999;20:495–9.
53. Jeyakumar A, Seth R, Brickman TM, et al. The prevalence and clinical course of patients with 'incidental' acoustic neuromas. Acta Otolaryngol 2007;127:1051–7.
54. Solares CA, Panizza B. Vestibular schwannoma: an understanding of growth should influence management decisions. Otol Neurotol 2008;29:829–34.
55. Hoa M, Drazin D, Hanna G, et al. The approach to the patient with incidentally diagnosed vestibular schwannoma. Neurosurg Focus 2012;33:1–7.
56. Stangerup SE, Thomsen J, Tos M, et al. Long-term hearing preservation in vestibular schwannoma. Otol Neurotol 2010;31:271–5.
57. Goddard JC, Schwartz MS, Friedman RA. Fundal fluid as a predictor of hearing preservation in the middle cranial fossa approach for vestibular schwannoma. Otol Neurotol 2010;31(7):1128–34.

Management of Sporadic Vestibular Schwannoma

Matthew L. Carlson, MD[a],*, Michael J. Link, MD[b,c], George B. Wanna, MD[d], Colin L.W. Driscoll, MD[b,c]

KEYWORDS

- Vestibular schwannoma • Acoustic neuroma • Cerebellopontine angle
- Internal auditory canal • Skull base

KEY POINTS

- The majority of patients with small to medium tumors experience high rates of tumor control and excellent facial nerve outcomes, regardless of treatment modality.
- At 10 years, less than a one-quarter of patients who started with serviceable hearing will maintain class A or B hearing regardless of the treatment modality employed.
- There is compelling evidence that, in the long term, patient-related factors are the primary drivers of quality of life, and treatment strategy has less impact.
- Long-term follow-up should be prioritized in vestibular schwannoma outcomes, where the majority of patients are expected to survive many decades beyond their diagnosis and treatment.
- Patients should receive individualized management based on personal priorities, health status, anticipated life expectancy, and symptoms.

INTRODUCTION

Understanding the history of vestibular schwannoma (VS) treatment is to know the development of modern lateral skull base surgery. VS is the model disease that defined a specialty, leading to the refinement of middle and posterior fossa skull base approaches, intraoperative cranial nerve monitoring, and collaboration between the neurotologist and neurosurgeon. The first surgeon to successfully remove a VS remains disputed secondary to uncertainties over tumor pathology, with either Charles Ballance in 1892 or Thomas Annandale in 1895 deserving credit.[1] The first significant breakthrough in the treatment of VS came with Cushing's introduction of

Financial and Material Support: No funding or other support was required for this study.
[a] Department of Otolaryngology-Head and Neck Surgery, Mayo Clinic School of Medicine, Mayo Clinic, 200 First Street Southwest, Rochester, MN 55905, USA; [b] Department of Otolaryngology-Head and Neck Surgery, Mayo Clinic School of Medicine, 200 First Street Southwest, Rochester, MN 55905, USA; [c] Department of Neurologic Surgery, Mayo Clinic School of Medicine, 200 First Street Southwest, Rochester, MN 55905, USA; [d] Department of Otolaryngology-Head and Neck Surgery, Vanderbilt University, Nashville, TN 37232, USA
* Corresponding author.
E-mail address: carlson.matthew@mayo.edu

oto.theclinics.com

the mastoid-to-mastoid bilateral suboccipital craniotomy with subtotal resection in place of finger enucleation, decreasing mortality from 80% to less than 20%.[2] Subsequently, Walter Dandy, Cushing's protégé and later rival, advocated a unilateral approach with complete tumor removal.[3,4]

In 1951, Swedish neurosurgeon, Lars Leksell introduced the concept of stereotactic radiosurgery (SRS) with the first VS treated in Stockholm with a fixed cobalt 60 source unit in 1969, citing the significant morbidity of surgery and Cushing's own reference to the need for noninvasive treatment methods.[5,6] Simultaneously, microsurgical advances came in the 1960s with William House and the adoption of the operating microscope and otologic drill, resulting in a further reduction in patient mortality and improved prospects of cranial nerve preservation with surgical removal of VS.[7,8] It was during this time that the middle fossa craniotomy and the translabyrinthine approaches were revisited after being abandoned for 6 decades because of technical limitations of the time.[9,10] The last significant advancement within the field of VS microsurgery came with the utilization of cranial nerve monitoring, first pioneered by Delgado and colleagues in 1979.[11]

Current management options for VS include observation with serial imaging, external beam radiation in the form of SRS (1–5 fractions) or stereotactic radiotherapy (>5 fractions), and microsurgical resection. Practically speaking, the viability of modern treatment modalities differ for small to medium tumors (<3 cm) compared with large VS; therefore, these 2 populations are usually discussed separately. In contrast with large tumors with problematic brainstem compression and symptoms of mass effect where surgery is strongly preferred, many smaller tumors can be managed effectively with observation, radiation, or microsurgical resection. Despite the significant volume of literature analyzing VS outcomes, the management of small to medium VS remains highly controversial. The fact that many VS centers are either dominated by SRS or microsurgery suggests that in most environments, provider bias remains the strongest factor dictating treatment. However, it also should be acknowledged that a number of patients seek out various centers with the intent of receiving a particular therapy. The remaining discussion is dedicated to understanding the advantages, limitations, and controversial aspects of the 3 available treatment modalities.

Microsurgery

Historically, and before the widespread availability of SRS, surgical resection was the preferred treatment for VS. The primary advantages of gross total surgical resection (GTR) include a high rate of long-term tumor control, improvement in symptoms of mass effect, definitive histopathologic confirmation of benign schwannoma, and potentially less intense imaging surveillance going forward. It is also sometimes presented that clinical outcomes of SRS after microsurgery, in cases of recurrence or less than GTR, are more favorable than microsurgery after SRS, in cases of continued tumor growth after radiation. This, in addition to the fact that recurrence after gross total resection is lower than reported SRS failure, is often used as an argument for microsurgery when all else is equal. Conversely, the primary disadvantages of surgery include a greater risk of permanent facial palsy, headache, treatment-related hearing loss, cerebrospinal fluid leak, meningitis, and very rarely stroke or death. Additionally microsurgery requires general anesthesia and a 3- to 5-day hospital stay on average with increased upfront cost, whereas SRS is performed with local anesthesia as an outpatient. Although somewhat controversial, frequently cited indications for primary microsurgery include younger patient age, larger tumor size with symptoms attributable to mass effect, ongoing dizziness, cystic tumors, and small anatomically favorable tumors with good hearing.[12]

Over the last 100 years, there have been a number of described surgical approaches to the internal auditory canal (IAC) and cerebellopontine angle (CPA); however, the retrosigmoid, translabyrinthine, and middle cranial fossa remain the most commonly used techniques today, each with their own merits and limitations.[1] The translabyrinthine approach was first described in 1904 by Panse, but was not popularized until the 1960s, paralleling the adoption of the operating microscope and drill to skull base surgery (**Fig. 1**).[9,13] The translabyrinthine craniotomy sacrifices hearing as a part of the operation and therefore is generally reserved for patients with nonserviceable hearing or cases where hearing preservation is not realistically feasible because of tumor size. The primary advantages of the translabyrinthine approach include minimal to no brain retraction, reliable distal identification of the facial nerve at the meatal foramen, and extradural drilling, which reduces subarachnoid bone dust dissemination and risk of intracranial injury from the rotating drill. Additionally, this approach best mitigates dizziness in patients presenting with vertigo and carries a lower risk of headaches than the retrosigmoid craniotomy, explained by minimal division of nuchal musculature and lack of intradural drilling.[14–17] Although some groups only use the translabyrinthine approach for smaller tumors, others report that, with modifications, tumor size is not a limiting factor. It has been our experience that the standard translabyrinthine approach can be more limiting than the retrosigmoid approach with very large tumors that extend far ventral to the porus acusticus, or with an unfavorable facial nerve course over the superior pole of a large tumor. Additionally, a view of the caudal aspect of a large VS can be problematic in the setting of a high jugular bulb. However, these limitations can often be overcome with additional retrosigmoid bony decompression, skeletonization of the jugular bulb, more extensive anterior IAC trough development, and patience with internal debulking, capsule infolding, and tumor mobilization.

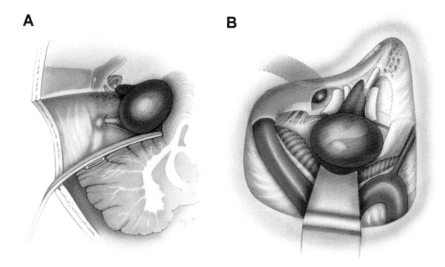

A   **B**

Fig. 1. (*A*) Axial view and (*B*) surgical vantage of the translabyrinthine approach for vestibular schwannoma resection. A retractor has been placed over the cerebellum, although this is not always used. Note the significant postsigmoid dural decompression performed to improve surgical exposure. Additionally, the meatal segment of the facial nerve can be readily identified early in dissection. (*Courtesy of* Christine Gralapp, MA, CMI, Fairfax, CA; with permission. Copyright © Chris Gralapp.)

The suboccipital approach for VS removal was first performed by Woolsey in 1903 and became popularized by Krause, followed by Cushing and Dandy years later.[2–4,18,19] The modern version of the retrosigmoid craniotomy is perhaps the most versatile of the 3 approaches, granting a panoramic view for removal of giant VS or the option for hearing preservation with small favorable medial tumors (**Fig. 2**). During hearing preservation, access to the lateral third of the IAC is limited by the position of the posterior semicircular canal and vestibule; however, view to the medial tumor in the cistern is uninhibited.[20] Some have reported the use of angled endoscopy for final inspection or disease removal at the fundus in cases of hearing preservation. It is helpful to carefully examine preoperative thinly sliced heavy T2 weighted sequences such as fast imaging employing steady-state acquisition (FIESTA) or constructive interference in steady state (CISS) to ascertain extent of tumor penetration within the IAC.

The choice between a retrosigmoid craniotomy or translabyrinthine approach for medium to large sized tumors for which hearing preservation is not a consideration, is often weighted toward surgeon preference. When versed in both approaches, the total operative time is not significantly different between the 2, with the main distinction being that meatal drilling and CPA access are performed before the tumor is engaged with the translabyrinthine approach, whereas IAC drilling is performed in a staged fashion after removing posterior fossa tumor during the retrosigmoid approach. Additionally, we have not noted a difference in facial nerve outcomes or risk of cerebrospinal fluid leak. The 2 theoretic drawbacks of the retrosigmoid craniotomy are the need for intradural drilling of the IAC and cerebellar retraction. Additionally, several studies have found that the risk of headaches is greater with retrosigmoid craniotomy than the translabyrinthine approach, particularly within the first postoperative year.[21]

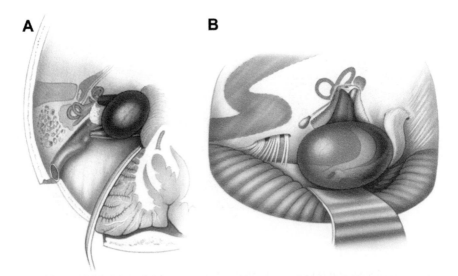

Fig. 2. (*A*) Axial view and (*B*) surgical vantage of the retrosigmoid approach for vestibular schwannoma resection. A retractor has been placed over the cerebellum. Note the broad view afforded by this approach, potentially from the foramen magnum to the tentorium cerebelli. (*Courtesy of* Christine Gralapp, MA, CMI, Fairfax, CA; with permission. Copyright © Chris Gralapp.)

The third and least commonly used approach is the middle fossa craniotomy (**Fig. 3**). This technique was first described by Parry in 1904 for vestibular nerve section, but was abandoned for approximately 60 years because of the severe morbidity associated with the inexact surgical techniques using unmagnified mallet and chisel bone removal.[10,22] In 1961, House revisited the middle fossa technique initially for removal of extensive otosclerosis, but soon realized its merits for IAC exposure for VS.[7] The middle fossa craniotomy uses extradural subtemporal access to the IAC and is primarily used for hearing preservation attempts with small, laterally based tumors. As a result of more limited access to the posterior fossa and because of poor prospects of hearing preservation with larger tumors, most surgeons limit tumor size to less than 0.5 cm in the CPA when considering a middle fossa approach. Although this point is often debated, proponents of the middle fossa craniotomy cite improved access to lateral tumor extent, compared with the retrosigmoid approach. The primary disadvantages of the middle cranial fossa approach are limited access to the posterior fossa and the need for temporal lobe retraction, which adds a very small risk of seizure, aphasia, and stroke. Additionally, because the IAC is accessed from above, the facial nerve position is often less optimal, requiring the surgeon to work around the nerve while removing tumor. Thus, when comparing tumors size and operative approach, the risk of facial paresis is greater with the middle fossa approach compared with others.[23,24] This has led some groups to perform preoperative vestibular testing and more detailed imaging studies to ascertain nerve of origin because, theoretically, tumors arising from the superior vestibular nerve are more favorable than inferior vestibular nerve tumors with regard to both the degree of facial nerve manipulation that may be required as well as risk to hearing and the

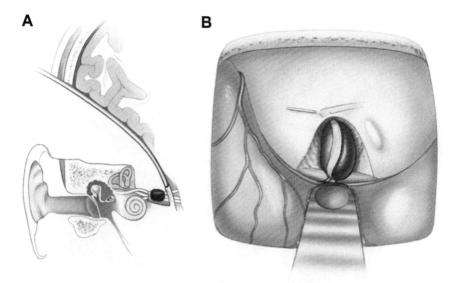

A   **B**

Fig. 3. (*A*) Coronal view and (*B*) surgical vantage of the middle fossa craniotomy for vestibular schwannoma resection. Note the retractor placement on the lip of the petrous ridge, over the temporal lobe. In this case, the meatal segment of the facial nerve can be seen coursing over top the tumor, a configuration that is less favorable for immediate postoperative facial nerve function. (*Courtesy of* Christine Gralapp, MA, CMI, Fairfax, CA; with permission. Copyright © Chris Gralapp.)

cochlear nerve. With vestibular testing, abnormal caloric testing may indicate a superior vestibular nerve tumor, whereas vestibular evoked myogenic potential results may be used to identify inferior vestibular nerve origin. However, once a tumor has reached a larger size, these methods of prediction become less reliable.

Stereotactic Radiotherapy

The concept of combining a stereotactic head frame with collimated x-ray beams was conceived by Lars Leksell of Sweden in 1951.[6] To date, the majority of the published outcomes for VS are from centers using the Leksell Gamma Knife system (Elekta AB, Stockholm, Sweden), incorporating a rigid head frame and between 192 (model Perfexion) and 201 (model U, B, C models) fixed sources of cobalt-60 (**Fig. 4**). During treatment planning, varying numbers of isocenters using different sized collimators, variably weighted, are used to create a radiation dose plan that highly conforms to the radiographic tumor volume on thin slice (1 mm) gadolinium enhanced MRI. The very steep radiation fall-off above the traditionally prescribed 50% isodose line results in a very conformal dose plan while minimizing dose to adjacent sensitive structures.

Early SRS series commonly used high-dose treatment plans (>16 Gy marginal dose) that achieved excellent tumor control (~98%); however, rates of early hearing loss, as well as facial and trigeminal neuropathy, were high. With time, several groups trialed dose de-escalation, to 13 and 14 Gy, and more recently 11 and 12 Gy, for patients with good pretreatment hearing.[25–27] At these levels, the risk of permanent facial palsy is less than 1% and more than 90% of patients still achieve durable tumor control. Clearly, at some point continuing to lower the dose to achieve better rates of hearing preservation will result in a noticeable decline in tumor control; however, at least in the sporadic VS population, this threshold has not yet been reached. Recently, minimizing cochlear dose during SRS to reduce the risk of hearing loss has become a popular topic. Until there is evidence that tumor control is achieved at much lower doses than 12 Gy, we believe that undertreating the lateral tumor margin to achieve a cochlear dose of less than 4 Gy is not advisable. It is clear that cochlear dose is only one of many factors that influence hearing decline after SRS.[28] In our center, we commonly use a marginal dose of 12.5 Gy prescribed to the 50% isodose line

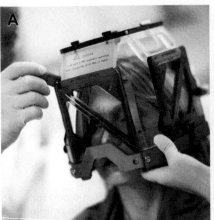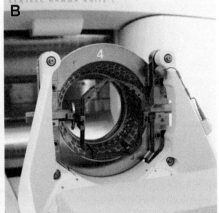

Fig. 4. (A) Leksell titanium head frame and (B) the Leksell GammaKnife Model 4C helmet housing 201 collimators, used in the radiosurgical treatment of vestibular schwannoma. (*Courtesy of* Elekta, Stockholm, Sweden; with permission.)

for patients with sporadic tumors and serviceable hearing and 13 to 14 Gy for patients with nonserviceable hearing. In our experience, tumor control is more problematic for patients with neurofibromatosis type 2, where we feel a higher dose paradigm is justified.[29]

Because the risk of immediate profound hearing loss after SRS is very low, this treatment was initially touted as a hearing preservation strategy. However, as our experience grows, it is clear that treatment at even lower marginal doses, such as 12 Gy, results in accelerated hearing loss. Several studies have documented surprisingly similar patterns of audiometric decline after SRS.[30–32] Within the first 2 years after treatment, there may be a rather steep drop in serviceable hearing, with a more shallow but steady decline thereafter.

One final aspect of SRS treatment that deserves review is the concern over radiation-induced malignancy. The modified Cahan criteria were established to help determine with reasonable probability whether a malignancy truly developed as a result of prior radiation rather than by chance or from an unrelated cause.[33] To date, there have been fewer than 10 radiation-associated malignancies reported in patients with VS.[34] Using the denominator of all patients treated worldwide, the risk of developing a radiation-induced cancer after SRS is less than 1 in 1000. It seems that this risk is greater in the neurofibromatosis type 2 population, where patients already harbor a mutation in a tumor suppressor gene.[35] One-half of radiation-associated malignancies occurring after SRS for VS have developed in neurofibromatosis type 2 patients; however, this group only represents 5% of the VS population. When interpreting these estimates, it is important to realize that the Cahan criteria are not perfect, because malignancy may occur coincidentally, even after microsurgery.[36] And because tissue biopsy is rarely performed before SRS, it is also possible that a small number of reported cases involving presumed VS were in fact malignancies all along. Regardless, to keep perspective, it is clear that the rate of radiation induced malignancy is extremely low in patients with sporadic VS, significantly below the lowest rates of mortality in surgical series from large experienced centers. Therefore, patients should be informed about this rare risk, but it should not be used to direct treatment.

Observation

Ironically, one of the greatest advances in VS management has been an understanding that many patients do not require treatment. Observing a central tenant of the skull base specialty, in the setting of benign disease, we should avoid inflicting more morbidity with treatment than the disease is expected to produce over the anticipated lifespan of the patient. In the early era of modern skull base surgery, the mere diagnosis of VS warranted aggressive tumor resection, prioritizing disease eradication even over facial nerve outcome. Beginning in the mid 1970s, several centers began adopting an expectant approach using a primary "wait-and-scan" policy for small tumors.[37] Particularly within the last 15 years, a growing number of publications characterizing the natural history of disease have emerged. Most studies have observed that more than 50% of intracanalicular tumors do not grow after diagnosis and a small percent actually regress.[37–39] Of course, because VS are not thought to be congenital lesions, every VS must enter a phase of growth to achieve the size seen at diagnosis; however, it seems that tumors may enter periods of extended or indefinite quiescence with time. To date, no consistent association between growth and tumor size or patient age have been identified. However, because the typical growth rate of enlarging tumors is 1 to 2 mm/y, observation poses extremely little risk to the patient, provided reliable follow-up can be maintained.

Perhaps the most controversial aspect of observation is the risk to hearing. Several studies have documented the long-term pattern of hearing loss in untreated tumors. These studies confirm that better hearing at diagnosis portends the greatest chance for long-term serviceable hearing.[40,41] The primary argument against observation is the belief that immediate or proactive treatment with SRS or microsurgery may protect useful long-term serviceable hearing, believing that waiting for growth reduces the success of hearing preservation treatment. For reasons outlined elsewhere in this article, the authors believe that overall, the greatest number of serviceable hearing years comes with observation compared with proactive treatment.

Undoubtedly, observation will become increasingly important in coming years with the growing number of small tumors diagnosed in patients with minimal attributable symptoms. Additionally, this strategy is appealing in the cost-consciousness climate of today. However, over a period of time the cumulative price of frequent MRI surveillance with observation may exceed the cost of early treatment. At the authors' centers, most patients with tumors less than 2 cm are observed initially and treatment is generally reserved for those with documented tumor growth.

COMPARISON OF TREATMENT MODALITIES BY TRADITIONAL MEASURES

Over the past 50 years, tumor control, facial nerve function, and hearing preservation have been the primary outcome measures of interest, evidenced by the disproportionately large number of publications focusing on these data. Understanding the natural history of untreated VS is paramount when discussing tumor control with SRS because a successful outcome is defined by a lack of growth, in contrast with surgery, where the goal of treatment is tumor removal. Several studies have demonstrated that overall less than one-half of conservatively followed VS demonstrate radiologic progression.[37–39] The rates of tumor control with SRS vary by series, but most centers report stable tumor volume or shrinkage in more than 90% of sporadic VS with varying lengths of follow-up. However, because many centers offer SRS without documented growth, this figure must be tempered by the fact that a proportion of these tumors were not destined to grow, so the actual rate of tumor control is likely lower.[42] Finally, the rate of tumor control after surgery must be evaluated by extent of resection, which has been defined inconsistently in the literature. In patients undergoing gross total resection, the risk of tumor recurrence is less than 3% in most series. When reviewing rates of residual progressive disease after less-than-complete resection, it is critical to evaluate how subtotal or near total resection is defined. Many authors have utilized a less than 95% volume cutoff to designate subtotal resection, and 95% to 99.9% volume range to define near-total resection. We believe this is problematic, because it is likely the absolute volume of residual tumor that predicts recurrence rather than the percentage of tumor volume; 5% of a 6 cm tumor is very large, whereas 5% of a 5 mm intracanalicular tumor is miniscule.[43,44] Similar to several other authors, we designate near total resection as leaving only a microscopic tumor capsule remnant (~5 × 2 × 2 mm or less) on the facial nerve or brainstem, and anything more is classified as subtotal resection.[43,45] Applying this definition, we found that the rate of recurrence after NTR was similar to GTR at approximately 3%; however, the risk of disease progression after subtotal resection is between 20% and 32%.[43,45] Thus, when comparing tumor control between treatment modalities, it is critical to evaluate study definitions and determine the treatment parameters of the study population.

The literature clearly demonstrates that the risk of permanent facial neuropathy is closely tied to method of treatment. Development of facial palsy during observation is exceptionally rare, and should raise suspicion for other less common pathologies, such as a facial nerve schwannoma or a more aggressive tumor variant.[46] Facial nerve outcome after SRS is primarily related to the prescribed dose to the tumor margin. Because the facial nerve is connected intimately to the tumor capsule, there is no effective method to shield the facial nerve from radiation. Up to 29% of patients experience transient or permanent facial palsy when doses of more than 16 Gy are used; however, with contemporary low doses, fewer than 1% of subjects develop lasting facial paresis.[25–27] Although the risk of facial paralysis is highest with surgery, many series from large volume centers demonstrate that more than 90% of patients retain normal or near-normal (HB I-II) function. The strongest predictor of facial nerve outcome during surgery is tumor size.[47–49] When comparing similar tumor sizes between approaches, the risk of long-term facial nerve dysfunction is not significantly different between the translabyrinthine and retrosigmoid craniotomy.[50,51] This is not surprising, because both are posterior fossa approaches having only a slightly different angle of access defined by position of the sigmoid sinus. In both approaches, the dorsal aspect of the tumor is debulked with the facial nerve coursing over the ventral face. This is in contrast with the middle fossa craniotomy, used primarily for hearing preservation of purely intracanalicular tumors, where the nerve is often immediately over or closely adjacent to the surgical corridor during tumor removal.[23]

One of the most controversial aspects of VS management is optimal treatment of patients presenting with smaller VS and serviceable hearing. There are a number of studies advocating early treatment with either microsurgery or SRS, believing that early proactive management offers the best chance of long-term serviceable hearing. The range of published outcomes for hearing preservation varies significantly between centers; however, the overall average after surgery is approximately 50%.[52] Several studies have demonstrated that, even if surgery is successful initially, hearing loss in the operated ear is still somewhat accelerated over normal physiologic loss.[53–55] The rate of audiometric decline after SRS has been documented in several recent studies, most of which demonstrate surprisingly consistent findings. Overall, at 5 years, approximately 50% of patients with pretreatment serviceable hearing will maintain class A or B hearing. At 10 years, this estimate decreases to approximately 25%.[30–32] Finally, the rate of hearing deterioration has been well-characterized by several natural history studies and is strongly tied with hearing levels at diagnosis. Among patients with class A or B hearing at time of diagnosis, 55% of patients retained serviceable hearing at 5 years. When examining only patients presenting with class A hearing at the time of diagnosis, 55% maintained class A hearing at 5 years, and 46% at 10 years.[56] Finally, in the most extreme example, 88% of tumors with 100% speech discrimination at the time of diagnosis will maintain good hearing for extended periods of time, compared with only 55% of those with less than 100% speech discrimination.[40]

When interpreting data on hearing preservation, there are several important points to consider. First, comparing the length of follow-up is critical, because duration since treatment is strongly associated with the development of nonserviceable hearing for all modalities. Second, the features that make a tumor favorable for 1 strategy also lend themselves to better outcomes with other management modalities. For example, very good pretreatment hearing capacity and small tumor size are strongly associated with a greater chance for hearing preservation in the microsurgery, SRS, and observation literature. Conversely, large tumors, fundal impaction or inner ear invasion, IAC erosion, and poor preoperative word discrimination predict poor outcomes independent of management strategy. It is also important to realize that there is likely considerable selection bias in surgical series. That is, hearing preservation is offered primarily to younger patients with smaller tumors and excellent hearing. Patients with medium to large tumors and patients with borderline serviceable hearing are less likely to be offered attempted hearing preservation and are more frequently excluded from these series. In contrast, centers commonly using early observation have a more inclusive population. Thus, when comparing all treatment modalities, even in a carefully selected patient group with an experienced surgeon, the early risk of deafness is likely greatest with microsurgery followed by SRS and observation.

Reviewing Nontraditional Outcome Measures

In an effort to further compare treatment modalities and refine patient outcomes, we have witnessed a growing number of publications evaluating other less tangible features, such as headache and dizziness, conditions that are more difficult to quantify, but are known to significantly influence patient well-being. In a recent study, we found that, when evaluating associations between various outcome parameters and disease-specific quality of life, ongoing dizziness and headache predicted the greatest reduction in quality of life, whereas facial palsy, hearing loss and tinnitus were less by comparison, a finding that is supported by several earlier studies.[57–60]

Traditionally, headache outcome reporting has been limited primarily to microsurgical series. Within this body of literature, it has been shown that the retrosigmoid approach is associated with a greater risk of problematic headaches after surgery, compared with middle fossa and translabyrinthine approaches.[23] There have been several proposed mechanisms for this outcome, including disseminated bone dust within the CPA from intradural meatal drilling, occipital nerve injury, division of nuchal musculature, and scar adhesion of neck muscle onto exposed dura.[14–17] Several studies have demonstrated a decrease in postoperative headache using craniotomy with bone flap replacement or cranioplasty compared with unreconstructed craniectomy.[15,17]

It is notable, however, that the apparent difference in headache outcomes between surgical approaches is no longer evident beyond 1 to 2 years postoperatively.[21] Even more interesting, the difference in long-term headache disability does not seem to be different between treatment modalities. In a recent publication evaluating headache disability at an average of approximately 8 years after treatment, there was no difference between patients receiving observation, SRS, and microsurgery using multivariable regression.[61] Instead, the primary predictors of poor long-term headache disability were younger age, preexisting headaches, and greater anxiety and depression. When examining the prevalence of posttreatment headache, it is important to consider that approximately one-half of the general population experience headaches and one-fifth suffer from migraines at baseline, and it is unlikely that treatment will make this better.[61] Thus, the clinician should be careful to examine for high-risk features at time of presentation to counsel the patient regarding long-term risk of severe headache. Furthermore, the presence of preexisting headaches should not necessarily steer treatment away from surgery given the nominal long-term differences between groups.

Despite the finding that dizziness is a ubiquitous complaint and consistently ranks among the most disabling of disease-related symptoms, this condition has received disproportionately little attention in the VS literature.[57,62] In a recent study examining long-term dizziness handicap in patients treated with microsurgery, SRS, and observation, pretreatment dizziness and ongoing posttreatment headaches were the strongest predictors of poor long-term dizziness outcomes; treatment strategy did not influence dizziness handicap outcome in a multivariable model.[62] Furthermore, symptoms of general unsteadiness were associated with greater handicap than vertigo and light headedness.

In patients with VS, it is generally assumed that vertigo is the result of vestibulopathy from eighth nerve compression or tumor involvement of the inner ear. Therefore, it is commonly held that vestibuloablative procedures (ie, surgery) offer the greatest chance for improvement by division of the eighth nerve or labyrinthectomy, providing a fixed deficit to accommodate to.[14,63] However, the growing body of literature suggests that long-term outcomes in patients with or without dizziness at the time of presentation are not different between treatment modalities. In fact, contrary to popular belief, there is often a trend toward surgery having slightly worse dizziness outcomes than SRS.[12,64] This can likely be explained by the fact that constant symptoms of complete ipsilateral vestibular hypofunction seem to be more problematic for most patients than episodic vertigo.[62] Because of these findings, we generally no longer dissuade patients from SRS or observation if they complain of severe dizziness at presentation.

Quality-of-Life Outcomes

Understanding that what physicians prioritize and what patients value may be different, health-related quality-of-life outcomes have gained increasing attention within the past 2 decades. Such data are particularly relevant to benign tumors such as VS, when disease-related mortality approaches zero and there are no large differences between available treatment outcomes based on traditional measures.

A significant limitation in the past has been the lack of a disease specific quality of life measure. As result, the general purpose Glasgow Benefit Inventory (GBI) and the 36-item Short Form Health Survey (SF36) have served as the default measures over the past 2 decades.[65,66] Although generic measures facilitate comparisons across different disease processes, they often lack the sensitivity necessary to detect subtle changes that occur as a result of disease or treatment, and are often significantly influenced by patient comorbidities. Recently, the Penn Acoustic Neuroma Quality of Life (PANQOL) scale was developed.[67] Compared with the SF36, and GBI, the PANQOL has proven a much more sensitive metric for comparing treatment modalities.[12,67]

To date, there have been only 3 prospective observational studies comparing quality of life between treatment modalities using general purpose measures and 2 cross-sectional observational studies using the PANQOL; currently, no level I evidence exists.[12,64,68–70] Summarizing the existing data, the majority of studies demonstrate very little long-term difference between treatment modalities. The few studies that have found significant differences generally only demonstrate a several point disparity on a 100-point scale, values that may not necessarily have real clinical significance.

SUMMARY

When performed by an experienced team, the majority of patients with small to medium tumors experience high rates of tumor control and excellent facial nerve outcomes, regardless of treatment modality. However, the long-term prospects of ipsilateral serviceable hearing are poor; at 10 years, fewer than one-quarter of patients who started with serviceable hearing maintain class A or B hearing regardless of the treatment modality employed. Despite short-term outcome data suggesting that certain treatment strategies or operative approaches are better than others at mitigating dizziness and headache, there is compelling evidence that, in the long term, patient-related factors are the primary drivers and treatment strategy has much less impact.[61,62] Finally, long-term quality-of-life outcome differences between treatment groups are very small.[12]

Unfortunately, few prospective studies exist and no randomized controlled trials comparing treatment modalities have been reported.[12,68–70] Furthermore, the median follow-up for most publications is short. This is particularly problematic when comparing microsurgery with radiosurgery or observation, because operative resection imparts early morbidity, whereas complications from SRS and untreated disease often accumulate over many years.[12] Long-term follow-up should be prioritized in VS outcomes, where the majority of patients are expected to survive many decades beyond their diagnosis and treatment. The best existing data suggest that there is currently not one supreme treatment. Rather, patients should receive individualized management based on personal priorities, health status, anticipated life expectancy, and, to a lesser degree, symptoms. Based on the natural history of VS, we as a profession are likely overtreating this disease.[71] Initial observation should be considered the default strategy for most patients with small tumors and minimal symptoms, because there is no clear advantage of upfront treatment in most cases.

REFERENCES

1. Ramsden RT. The bloody angle: 100 years of acoustic neuroma surgery. J R Soc Med 1995;88(8):464P–8P.
2. Cushing H. Tumors of the nervus acusticus and the syndrome of the cerbellopontile angle. Philadelphia: W.B. Saunders Company; 1917.
3. Dandy WE. Removal of cerebellopontine tumors through a unilateral approach. Arch Surg 1934;29:337–44.
4. Dandy WE. An operation for the total removal of cerebellpontile tumors. Surg Gynecol Obstet 1925;41:129.
5. Leksell L. A note on the treatment of acoustic tumours. Acta Chir Scand 1971; 137(8):763–5.
6. Leksell L. The stereotaxic method and radiosurgery of the brain. Acta Chir Scand 1951;102(4):316–9.
7. House WF. Middle cranial fossa approach to the petrous pyramid. Report of 50 cases. Arch Otolaryngol 1963;78:460–9.
8. House WF. Transtemporal bone microsurgical removal of acoustic neuromas. Evolution of transtemporal bone removal of acoustic tumors. Arch Otolaryngol 1964;80:731–42.
9. Panse R. Klinische und pathologische Mitteilungen. IV. Ein Gliom des Akustikus. Archiv Ohrenh 1904;61:251–5.
10. Parry RH. A case of tinnitus and vertigo treated by division of the auditory nerve. J Laryngol Otol 1904;19:402.
11. Delgado TE, Bucheit WA, Rosenholtz HR, et al. Intraoperative monitoring of facila muscle evoked responses obtained by intracranial stimulation of the facila nerve: a more accurate technique for facila nerve dissection. Neurosurgery 1979;4(5): 418–21.
12. Carlson M, Tveiten Ø, Driscoll C, et al. Long-term quality of life in patients with vestibular schwannoma: an international multicenter, cross-sectional study comparing microsurgery, stereotactic radiosurgery, observation, and non-tumor controls. J Neurosurg 2015. [Epub ahead of print]
13. Nguyen-Huynh AT, Jackler RK, Pfister M, et al. The aborted early history of the translabyrinthine approach: a victim of suppression or technical prematurity? Otol Neurotol 2007;28(2):269–79.
14. Godefroy WP, Hastan D, van der Mey AG. Translabyrinthine surgery for disabling vertigo in vestibular schwannoma patients. Clin Otolaryngol 2007;32(3):167–72.

15. Harner SG, Beatty CW, Ebersold MJ. Impact of cranioplasty on headache after acoustic neuroma removal. Neurosurgery 1995;36(6):1097–9 [discussion: 1099–100].
16. Jackson CG, McGrew BM, Forest JA, et al. Comparison of postoperative headache after retrosigmoid approach: vestibular nerve section versus vestibular schwannoma resection. Am J Otol 2000;21(3):412–6.
17. Koperer H, Deinsberger W, Jodicke A, et al. Postoperative headache after the lateral suboccipital approach: craniotomy versus craniectomy. Minim Invasive Neurosurg 1999;42(4):175–8.
18. Fraenkel J, Hunt J, Woolsey G, et al. Contributions to the surgery of neurfibroma of the acoustic nerve with remarks on the surgical procedure. Ann Surg 1904;40: 293–319.
19. Krause E. Zur Freilegung der Linteren, Felsenbeinflache und des Kleinhirns, Beitr 2. Kline Chir 1903;XXXVII:728–64.
20. Blevins NH, Jackler RK. Exposure of the lateral extremity of the internal auditory canal through the retrosigmoid approach: a radioanatomic study. Otolaryngol Head Neck Surg 1994;111(1):81–90.
21. Ruckenstein MJ, Harris JP, Cueva RA, et al. Pain subsequent to resection of acoustic neuromas via suboccipital and translabyrinthine approaches. Am J Otol 1996;17(4):620–4.
22. Monfared A, Mudry A, Jackler R. The history of middle cranial fossa approach to the cerebellopontine angle. Otol Neurotol 2010;31(4):691–6.
23. Ansari SF, Terry C, Cohen-Gadol AA. Surgery for vestibular schwannomas: a systematic review of complications by approach. Neurosurg Focus 2012;33(3): E14.
24. Rabelo de Freitas M, Russo A, Sequino G, et al. Analysis of hearing preservation and facial nerve function for patients undergoing vestibular schwannoma surgery: the middle cranial fossa approach versus the retrosigmoid approach–personal experience and literature review. Audiol Neurootol 2012;17(2):71–81.
25. Flickinger JC, Lunsford LD, Linskey ME, et al. Gamma knife radiosurgery for acoustic tumors: multivariate analysis of four year results. Radiother Oncol 1993;27(2):91–8.
26. Flickinger JC, Kondziolka D, Lunsford LD. Dose and diameter relationships for facial, trigeminal, and acoustic neuropathies following acoustic neuroma radiosurgery. Radiother Oncol 1996;41(3):215–9.
27. Lunsford LD, Niranjan A, Flickinger JC, et al. Radiosurgery of vestibular schwannomas: summary of experience in 829 cases. J Neurosurg 2013;119(Suppl): 195–9.
28. Jacob JT, Carlson ML, Schiefer TK, et al. Significance of cochlear dose in the radiosurgical treatment of vestibular schwannoma: controversies and unanswered questions. Neurosurgery 2014;74(5):466–74 [discussion: 474].
29. Mallory GW, Pollock BE, Foote RL, et al. Stereotactic radiosurgery for neurofibromatosis 2-associated vestibular schwannomas: toward dose optimization for tumor control and functional outcomes. Neurosurgery 2014;74(3):292–300 [discussion: 300–1].
30. Carlson ML, Jacob JT, Pollock BE, et al. Long-term hearing outcomes following stereotactic radiosurgery for vestibular schwannoma: patterns of hearing loss and variables influencing audiometric decline. J Neurosurg 2013;118(3):579–87.
31. Roos DE, Potter AE, Zacest AC. Hearing preservation after low dose linac radiosurgery for acoustic neuroma depends on initial hearing and time. Radiother Oncol 2011;101(3):420–4.

32. Hasegawa T, Kida Y, Kato T, et al. Factors associated with hearing preservation after Gamma Knife surgery for vestibular schwannomas in patients who retain serviceable hearing. J Neurosurg 2011;115(6):1078–86.

33. Cahan WG, Woodard HQ, Higinbotham NL, et al. Sarcoma arising in irradiated bone; report of 11 cases. Cancer 1948;1(1):3–29.

34. Schmitt WR, Carlson ML, Giannini C, et al. Radiation-induced sarcoma in a large vestibular schwannoma following stereotactic radiosurgery: case report. Neurosurgery 2011;68(3):E840–6 [discussion: E846].

35. Carlson ML, Babovic-Vuksanovic D, Messiaen L, et al. Radiation-induced rhabdomyosarcoma of the brainstem in a patient with neurofibromatosis type 2. J Neurosurg 2010;112(1):81–7.

36. Hoa M, Rhiew R, Kupsky WJ, et al. Glioblastoma multiforme after microsurgery for acoustic neuroma without radiotherapy: limitations of the Cahan criteria. Otolaryngol Head Neck Surg 2008;139(2):323–4.

37. Stangerup SE, Caye-Thomasen P, Tos M, et al. The natural history of vestibular schwannoma. Otol Neurotol 2006;27(4):547–52.

38. Godefroy WP, Kaptein AA, Vogel JJ, et al. Conservative treatment of vestibular schwannoma: a follow-up study on clinical and quality-of-life outcome. Otol Neurotol 2009;30(7):968–74.

39. Selesnick SH, Johnson G. Radiologic surveillance of acoustic neuromas. Am J Otol 1998;19(6):846–9.

40. Stangerup SE, Caye-Thomasen P, Tos M, et al. Change in hearing during 'wait and scan' management of patients with vestibular schwannoma. J Laryngol Otol 2008;122(7):673–81.

41. Caye-Thomasen P, Dethloff T, Hansen S, et al. Hearing in patients with intracanalicular vestibular schwannomas. Audiol Neurootol 2007;12(1):1–12.

42. Miller T, Lau T, Vasan R, et al. Reporting success rates in the treatment of vestibular schwannomas: are we accounting for the natural history? J Clin Neurosci 2014;21(6):914–8.

43. Carlson ML, Van Abel KM, Driscoll CL, et al. Magnetic resonance imaging surveillance following vestibular schwannoma resection. Laryngoscope 2012;122(2):378–88.

44. Vakilian S, Souhami L, Melancon D, et al. Volumetric measurement of vestibular schwannoma tumour growth following partial resection: predictors for recurrence. J Neurol Surg B Skull Base 2012;73(2):117–20.

45. Bloch DC, Oghalai JS, Jackler RK, et al. The fate of the tumor remnant after less-than-complete acoustic neuroma resection. Otolaryngol Head Neck Surg 2004;130(1):104–12.

46. Espahbodi M, Carlson ML, Fang TY, et al. Small vestibular schwannomas presenting with facial nerve palsy. Otol Neurotol 2014;35(5):895–8.

47. Moffat DA, Parker RA, Hardy DG, et al. Factors affecting final facial nerve outcome following vestibular schwannoma surgery. J Laryngol Otol 2014;128(5):406–15.

48. Falcioni M, Fois P, Taibah A, et al. Facial nerve function after vestibular schwannoma surgery. J Neurosurg 2011;115(4):820–6.

49. Jacob A, Robinson LL Jr, Bortman JS, et al. Nerve of origin, tumor size, hearing preservation, and facial nerve outcomes in 359 vestibular schwannoma resections at a tertiary care academic center. Laryngoscope 2007;117(12):2087–92.

50. Gurgel RK, Dogru S, Amdur RL, et al. Facial nerve outcomes after surgery for large vestibular schwannomas: do surgical approach and extent of resection matter? Neurosurg Focus 2012;33(3):E16.

51. Ho SY, Hudgens S, Wiet RJ. Comparison of postoperative facial nerve outcomes between translabyrinthine and retrosigmoid approaches in matched-pair patients. Laryngoscope 2003;113(11):2014–20.
52. Sughrue ME, Yang I, Aranda D, et al. Hearing preservation rates after microsurgical resection of vestibular schwannoma. J Clin Neurosci 2010;17(9):1126–9.
53. Nakamizo A, Mori M, Inoue D, et al. Long-term hearing outcome after retrosigmoid removal of vestibular schwannoma. Neurol Med Chir 2013;53(10):688–94.
54. Wang AC, Chinn SB, Than KD, et al. Durability of hearing preservation after microsurgical treatment of vestibular schwannoma using the middle cranial fossa approach. J Neurosurg 2013;119(1):131–8.
55. Shelton C, Hitselberger WE, House WF, et al. Hearing preservation after acoustic tumor removal: long-term results. Laryngoscope 1990;100(2 Pt 1):115–9.
56. Stangerup SE, Thomsen J, Tos M, et al. Long-term hearing preservation in vestibular schwannoma. Otol Neurotol 2010;31(2):271–5.
57. Carlson M, Driscoll C, Neff B, et al. Quality-of-life comparing observation, microsurgery, and radiosurgery for small-to-medium sized vestibular schwannoma using a validated disease-specific instrument, in 23rd North American Skull Base Society Annual Meeting. Miami (FL), February 16, 2013.
58. Breivik CN, Varughese JK, Wentzel-Larsen T, et al. Conservative management of vestibular schwannoma–a prospective cohort study: treatment, symptoms, and quality of life. Neurosurgery 2012;70(5):1072–80 [discussion: 1080].
59. Varughese JK, Breivik CN, Wentzel-Larsen T, et al. Growth of untreated vestibular schwannoma: a prospective study. J Neurosurg 2012;116(4):706–12.
60. Lloyd SK, Kasbekar AV, Baguley DM, et al. Audiovestibular factors influencing quality of life in patients with conservatively managed sporadic vestibular schwannoma. Otol Neurotol 2010;31(6):968–76.
61. Carlson ML, Tveiten OV, Driscoll CL, et al. Risk factors and analysis of long-term headache in sporadic vestibular schwannoma: a multicenter cross-sectional study. J Neurosurg 2015. [Epub ahead of print]
62. Carlson ML, Tveiten OV, Driscoll CL, et al. Long-term dizziness handicap in patients with vestibular schwannoma: a multicenter cross-sectional study. Otolaryngol Head Neck Surg 2014;151(6):1028–37.
63. Giannuzzi AL, Merkus P, Falcioni M. The use of intratympanic gentamicin in patients with vestibular schwannoma and disabling vertigo. Otol Neurotol 2013; 34(6):1096–8.
64. Robinett ZN, Walz PC, Miles-Markley B, et al. Comparison of Long-term Quality-of-Life Outcomes in Vestibular Schwannoma Patients. Otolaryngol Head Neck Surg 2014;150(6):1024–32.
65. Gauden A, Weir P, Hawthorne G, et al. Systematic review of quality of life in the management of vestibular schwannoma. J Clin Neurosci 2011;18(12):1573–84.
66. Gouveris HT, Mann WJ. Quality of life in sporadic vestibular schwannoma: a review. ORL J Otorhinolaryngol Relat Spec 2010;72(2):69–74.
67. Shaffer BT, Cohen MS, Bigelow DC, et al. Validation of a disease-specific quality-of-life instrument for acoustic neuroma: the Penn acoustic neuroma quality-of-life scale. Laryngoscope 2010;120(8):1646–54.
68. Di Maio S, Akagami R. Prospective comparison of quality of life before and after observation, radiation, or surgery for vestibular schwannomas. J Neurosurg 2009;111(4):855–62.
69. Myrseth E, Moller P, Pedersen PH, et al. Vestibular schwannoma: surgery or gamma knife radiosurgery? A prospective, nonrandomized study. Neurosurgery 2009;64(4):654–61 [discussion: 661–3].

70. Pollock BE, Driscoll CL, Foote RL, et al. Patient outcomes after vestibular schwannoma management: a prospective comparison of microsurgical resection and stereotactic radiosurgery. Neurosurgery 2006;59(1):77–85 [discussion: 77–85].

71. Lau T, Olivera R, Miller T Jr, et al. Paradoxical trends in the management of vestibular schwannoma in the United States. J Neurosurg 2012;117(3):514–9.

Intralabyrinthine Schwannomas

Christopher D. Frisch, MD[a], Laurence J. Eckel, MD[b], Jack I. Lane, MD[b], Brian A. Neff, MD[a],*

KEYWORDS

- Intralabyrinthine schwannoma • Vestibular schwannoma • Acoustic neuroma
- Inner ear • Cochlea • Vestibule

KEY POINTS

- Most patients with intralabyrinthine schwannomas (ILS) will present with unilateral, severe sensorineural hearing loss as the primary indication to obtain an MRI.
- The differential diagnosis is predominately radiographic because hearing loss and vestibular symptoms are common to both ILS and other inner ear lesions.
- Interval MRI scanning and observation is currently performed for most patients with ILS, especially those without vestibular complaints.
- Surgical removal of ILS can be safely performed, and surgery may be increasingly indicated if cochlear implantation demonstrates effectiveness for unilateral hearing loss rehabilitation.

INTRODUCTION

Vestibular schwannomas are benign, slow-growing tumors that most commonly arise from the vestibular division of the eighth cranial nerve.[1,2] They account for approximately 80% to 90% of tumors within the cerebellopontine angle (CPA) and approximately 6% of all intracranial tumors.[3] Although there is ongoing debate over the specifics of tumor origin, most would agree that they arise from Schwann cells within the internal auditory canal (IAC). These progenitor Schwann cells are also found beyond the confines of the IAC in the more distal inner ear labyrinth.[4] Tumors arising in this area are far less common than the typical schwannoma involving the IAC. First described by Mayer[5] in 1917, the most recent systematic review of the literature revealed 234 intralabyrinthine schwannomas (ILS), which have now been described.[6]

Financial and Material Support: No funding or other support was required for this study.
Conflict of Interest to Declare: The authors report no conflicts of interest concerning the information presented in this paper.
The following article has not been previously published or submitted elsewhere for review.
[a] Department of Otolaryngology-Head and Neck Surgery, Mayo Clinic, 200 First Street Southwest, Rochester, MN 55905, USA; [b] Department of Radiology, Mayo Clinic, 200 First Street Southwest, Rochester, MN 55905, USA
* Corresponding author.
E-mail address: neff.brian@mayo.edu

Otolaryngol Clin N Am 48 (2015) 423–441
http://dx.doi.org/10.1016/j.otc.2015.02.004
0030-6665/15/$ – see front matter © 2015 Elsevier Inc. All rights reserved.

Before the advent of MRI, these tumors were found exclusively at the time of autopsy or as an unexpected discovery during neurotologic surgery for another reason, such as labyrinthectomy for Ménière disease.[7] Because of their rarity and presentation overlap with Ménière disease, diagnosis can be delayed. Visualizing these tumors is also a challenge because the MRI quality and sequences used are critical in avoiding a missed diagnosis.

ANATOMY AND PATHOGENESIS
Anatomy

The otic capsule is a dense section of bone within the petrous pyramid that houses the inner ear organs of hearing and balance. Collectively termed the membranous labyrinth, this includes the cochlea, semicircular canals, utricle, saccule, and endolymphatic duct and sac. The radiographic and surgical bony space that contains the utricle and saccule is called the vestibule. The bony labyrinth, containing perilymph, surrounds the more interior membranous portion, which contains endolymph. The neuroepithelium, which is responsible for this sensory system, is contained within the membranous portion.

The cochlea spirals 2 and a half times around a cone-shaped structure of porous bone called the modiolus, with the apex of the cone corresponding to the apex of the cochlea. The basilar membrane essentially separates the cochlea into a double-lumen tube made up of the scala tympani and scala vestibuli (**Fig. 1**). The scala tympani communicates with the middle ear near its basal turn via the round window. The scala tympani also connects to the posterior fossa via a potential space called the cochlear aqueduct, which, if abnormally enlarged, can be an open connection

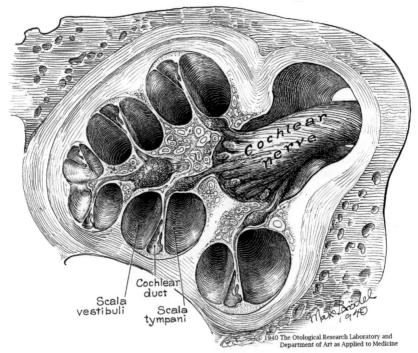

Cochlear nerve

Cochlear duct

Scala vestibuli

Scala tympani

© 1940 The Otological Research Laboratory and Department of Art as Applied to Medicine

Fig. 1. Anatomy of the cochlea and cochlear scalae. (Original illustration #9987 in the Walters Collection of the Max Brödel Archives. Department of Art as Applied to Medicine, The Johns Hopkins University School of Medicine, Baltimore, MD, USA. Used with permission.)

between the perilymph of the inner ear and cerebrospinal fluid (CSF). The scala media, or the cochlear duct, is an endolymph-containing portion of the membranous labyrinth that connects to the saccule via the ductus reuniens.

Within the modiolus are numerous bony canals called the Rosenthal canals, which are adjacent to the scala tympani and contain the spiral ganglia. The afferent branches of the cochlear nerve originate between the hair cells and the spiral ganglia. These nerve endings pierce the organ of Corti through multiple small openings called the habenula perforata. It is at this most distal location where Schwann cell myelination terminates. The afferent branches then run from the spiral ganglia through multiple small openings at the distal IAC called the cribriform plate. Just proximal to Scarpa's ganglion and just distal to the cribriform plate is the Schwann-glial cell junction of the cochlear division of the eighth cranial nerve.[8]

The bony vestibule, located between the cochlea and 3 semicircular canals, contains the utricle and saccule. The ampulated ends of the semicircular canals open into the utricle. The saccule communicates with the scala media of the cochlea via the ductus reuniens. Two small ducts, one each from the saccule and utricle, unite to form the endolymphatic duct. As its name implies, this endolymph-containing duct is also part of the membranous labyrinth and is housed within the bony vestibular aqueduct. The afferent nerve fibers traveling from the vestibular hair cells of the semicircular canals, utricle, and saccule pierce the cribriform plate of the distal IAC en route to the Scarpa's ganglia within the IAC. Unlike the cochlear division, the Schwann-glial cell junction of the vestibular divisions is at the Scarpa's ganglia (**Fig. 2**).[9] With this anatomy in mind, it is helpful to refer to the revised Kennedy classification system in order to describe tumor locations (**Fig. 3**).

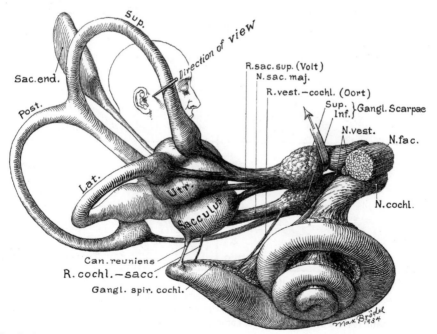

Fig. 2. Anatomy of the membranous labyrinth. (Original illustration #933 in the Walters Collection of the Max Brödel Archives. Department of Art as Applied to Medicine, The Johns Hopkins University School of Medicine, Baltimore, MD, USA. Used with permission.)

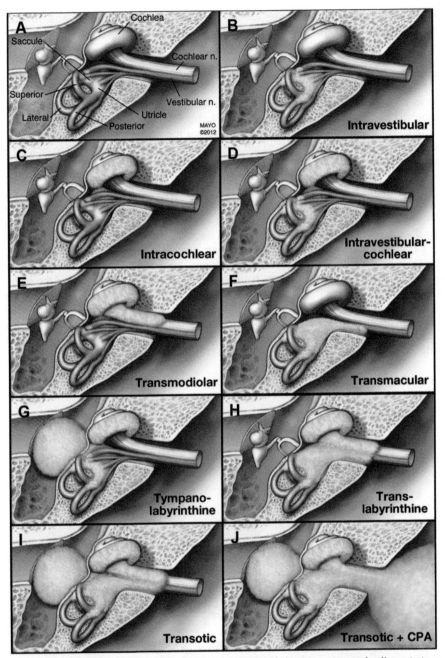

Fig. 3. Modified Kennedy classification. (*A*) Anatomy of the inner ear and adjacent structures. (*B–J*) Extent of tumor involvement for each subtype is depicted in yellow. (*From* Van Abel KV, Carlson ML, Link MJ, et al. Primary inner ear schwannomas: a case series and systematic review of the literature. Laryngoscope 2013;123(8):1959; with permission.)

Pathogenesis

Originally, it was thought that ILS occurred mainly in patients with neurofibromatosis type 2 (NF2).[10] However, more recent reviews have shown that the overall number of sporadic cases far outnumber NF2 cases because of the rarity of the latter. The genetics of sporadic ILS are not thought to be different from the more common vestibular schwannoma of the IAC and CPA, although confirmatory studies are still needed. ILS probably occur following 2 separate sporadic mutations within the *NF2* tumor suppressor gene; however, the location of the Schwann cells harboring the mutation is located distally within the inner ear. Schwann cells occur in higher density within the IAC near the Schwann-glial junction (Obersteiner-Redlich zone); controversially, this is thought by some to be the site of origin of the more common vestibular schwannoma of the IAC and CPA.[11,12] Similarly, it has been hypothesized that cochlear ILS might originate in the more distal cochlear nerve Schwann-glial junction in the modiolus, where Schwann cell concentration is also high.[6]

As is discussed further in the clinical presentation section, these tumors can cause variable symptoms depending on location of origin as well as pathway of growth. As postulated earlier, it is possible that most of these tumors originate in the terminal Schwann cells of the modiolus and then easily grow directly into the cochlea. This point could explain why the cochlea, specifically the basal turn, is the most common location for ILS, with many reports of tumors isolated to the modiolus or basal turn of the cochlea.[6,13–16] Lastly, the anatomy is relevant in terms of adjacent spaces into which these tumors may spread, thus influencing their presentation. Tumor spread is likely to occur along the path of least resistance and, therefore, is unlikely to spread beyond the highly dense otic capsule. However, the tumor can easily spread throughout the labyrinth: from cochlea to vestibule to semicircular canal and vice versa. Reports of tumors spreading to the middle ear by passing through the round window or displacing the stapes footplate are relatively rare.[17,18] Although not occurring frequently, the tumor may break through the cribriform plate located at the distal end of the IAC and then grow more proximally toward the CPA.

CLINICAL PRESENTATION

The average age for ILS diagnosis is 49 years (range 14–89 years), with no male-female predilection. Because of the relative rarity, overlap with other diagnoses, and difficult radiologic detection, the current average delay until diagnosis is around 7 years.[6] As alluded to previously, the overlap in ILS symptoms with other more common neurotologic diseases, such as Ménière disease, vestibular migraine, and vestibular schwannoma of the IAC and CPA, makes diagnosis challenging. As the most common symptoms are hearing loss and vertigo, the authors examine these in greatest detail in this section.

Hearing Loss

Early reports of ILS series demonstrated that nearly all patients initially presented with hearing loss.[1,7,19] In 2013, a large literature review examined 234 ILS and reported a 99% rate of hearing loss, with most cases (87%) presenting with American Academy of Otolaryngology–Head and Neck Surgery (AAO-HNS) class D hearing.[6,20] The pattern of hearing loss is variable and may not provide a means of discriminating these tumors from patients with Ménière disease. ILS have presented with progressive, sudden, and fluctuating patterns of hearing loss. One case series found rates of 61% progressive loss, 32% sudden loss, and 7% fluctuating hearing loss.[1] Another systematic review showed that fluctuating hearing loss occurred only 3% of the time for ILS, whereas many patients with ILS (39%) were misdiagnosed with Ménière disease.[6]

Although there have been histologic reports of isolated neural damage at only the tumor site, potentially causing isolated frequencies of hearing loss, this presentation is not seen in many ILS. The fact that many ILS do not involve the cochlea (30%), yet 99% of patients report hearing loss means other pathophysiologic mechanisms of hearing loss must exist. One hypothesis is that isolated tumors of the vestibule and semicircular canals still may cause hearing loss by either direct compression of the ductus reuniens or any other site along the pathway of endolymph flow toward the endolymphatic sac, thus leading to endolymphatic hydrops.[1] Others think that the presence of abnormal metabolites or interruption of potassium cycling within the tumor-containing labyrinth may directly damage or alter the function of the organ of Corti.[21,22]

Lastly, the clinician should be aware of the possibility of a mixed hearing loss occurring in a small subset of patients with ILS. Stapes footplate fixation or displacement into the middle ear from extension of intracochlear tumors can occur.[18,23] Hamed and Linthicum[24] captured an example of this in a temporal bone histology section of the cochlea and stapes footplate. In this patient, tumor was discovered filling the vestibule, primarily, but had extended into the proximal scala vestibuli. The tumor extended along the superior vestibular nerve as far as its entry point into the IAC but abruptly stopped at that point. Instead of growing into the IAC, stapes footplate dislocation into the middle ear had occurred. These examples of inner ear conductive hearing loss would appear as a mixed pattern on audiologic testing.

Vertigo and Disequilibrium

Patients with ILS may describe variable vestibular symptoms, including vertigo, motion-induced dizziness, and disequilibrium. Abnormal balance and unsteadiness were found to be more common than vertigo.[6] Vertigo has been reported in 59% of patients; the vertigo was episodic in all but 1 patient, who described constant vertigo. The relatively high rate of episodic vertigo described by these patients, in addition to the near-uniform presence of sensorineural hearing loss (SNHL) and tinnitus, makes differentiating these lesions from Ménière disease challenging.

The pathophysiologic mechanism to explain episodic vertigo is not definitively established. A greater rate of vestibular subsite involvement has been reported in patients presenting with vestibular symptoms, but vertigo can also occur with isolated cochlear lesions.[6] One report found that 26% (7 of 27) of patients with vertigo had isolated cochlear ILS. One possible explanation for why this occurs was hypothesized from temporal bone examinations. Three of 7 patients with cochlear ILS had histologic evidence of endolymphatic hydrops, and perhaps this is the reason for vestibular symptoms in patients having isolated cochlear involvement.[7]

Lastly, it should be noted that the percentage of patients with ILS having vertiginous symptoms seems to be higher than that of patients with the more common vestibular schwannoma of the IAC in whom the presentation is often disequilibrium without vertigo.[7] This higher rate might be because ILS arise from a more distal site within the vestibular system. Distal vestibular damage might create abnormal or fluctuating neural input to the more proximal vestibular system, whereas IAC schwannoma originating near Scarpa's ganglion might lead to a more stable, yet reduced, vestibular input to the brain stem.

Physical Findings

In general, physical examination findings in patients with intralabyrinthine tumors are rare, and most are nonspecific. For example, patients with unsteadiness or imbalance may have a positive Romberg test or may have gait instability on ambulatory testing. A patient experiencing an episodic flare of vertigo may have nystagmus. There are isolated reports of tumors presenting as a middle-ear mass and one reaching as far as the external auditory canal (**Fig. 4**).[17,18,25,26] In most patients, physical examination findings are lacking.

IMAGING

The diagnosis of an ILS is ultimately made with MRI in the context of the clinical presentation. Unfortunately, there are no pathognomonic clinical symptoms, physical examination findings, or audiologic criteria that will definitively suggest the presence of an ILS. Before the routine use of MRI for evaluation of inner ear and retrocochlear pathology, computed tomography (CT) was occasionally used but was often not helpful because of poor soft tissue resolution or lack of specificity in evaluating the labyrinth and IAC. There have been isolated reports of successful CT use in preoperatively diagnosing ILS but several others reporting their failure.[27–30] CT findings have been described as soft tissue masses within the cochlea with absence of the normal radiolucency within the basal turn.[31] Without bone erosion, or extension into the IAC or middle ear, the use of CT to diagnose ILS is limited.

Doyle and Brackmann[19] published their results of a series of 8 patients in whom MRI was used for preoperative diagnosis in all patients. They suggested MRI for preoperative localization and surgical planning or as a method of following the growth of stable tumors. Subsequently, there have been several published reports on the MRI findings of ILS. Many describe a lack of normal fluid density on T2-weighted imaging, with corresponding enhancement seen on gadolinium-enhanced T1-weighted scans.[9] However, other specific MRI sequences are also important for accurate diagnosis. The standard 2-dimensional (2D) fast-spin T2 sequence, typically acquired at a slice thickness of 3 mm, may miss smaller tumors.[6] Three-dimensional (3D) imaging techniques to include constructive interference in a steady state (3D CISS) and variable flip-angle 3D fast spin echo T2-weighted sequences (T2 SPACE), acquired at a 1-mm slice thickness or less, have become critical for the evaluation of pathology involving the membranous labyrinth and inner ear.[32] At the authors' institution, they also use variable flip-angle 3D fast spin echo (FSE) T1-weighted sequences (T1 SPACE), which can be acquired at 0.6-mm sections through the labyrinth. Using both the 3D T2-weighted sequences and fat-saturated postgadolinium 3D T1-weighted images allows for precise localization of tumor margins.[33] Physicians evaluating for ILS must make sure these sequences are performed because many routine MRI protocols may not include these sequences unless they are specifically requested.

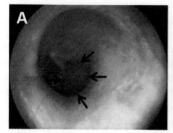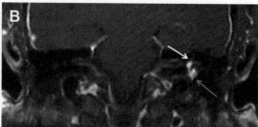

Fig. 4. (*A*) Otoscopic view of left ear. The posterior inferior mesotympanum shows a tan mass touching the tympanic membrane (*black arrows*). This mass is an ILS that has extended into the middle ear. (*B*) A coronal contrast-enhanced T1-weighted MRI showing the same left-sided ILS filling the vestibule (*white arrow*) and extending into the middle ear via the round window (*gray arrow*).

OTHER TESTING
Audiology

ILS can cause a variety of hearing loss patterns depending on the tumor size and location. Most patients present with a gradual-onset, severe or profound, unilateral SNHL. However, certain frequencies may rarely be spared with isolated cochlear tumors confined to the basal turn.[4] Fluctuating, low-frequency SNHL typical of endolymphatic hydrops or Ménière disease may be seen in a minority of patients with ILS. Sudden SNHL has also been reported at initial presentation.[19] Patients may rarely have a mixed hearing loss if the tumor causes an inner ear conductive loss.[23] Word recognition scores can be highly variable but are usually poor.[19]

Vestibular Testing

Although nonspecific, the use of vestibular testing, such as videonystagmography (VNG), rotary chair, or vestibular evoked myogenic potential, can be done for the evaluation of these patients. Decreased or completely absent responses on VNG may be seen. One small ILS case series found variable degrees of VNG vestibular hypofunction, seemingly dependent on the tumor location. Alternatively, one of their patients demonstrated significantly decreased vestibular response from an isolated cochlea and distal IAC tumor.[19] Other reports of abnormal vestibular testing in isolated cochlear tumors exist.[9,13]

Differential Diagnosis: Clinical and Radiographic

The clinical differential diagnosis of ILS depends on whether the patient is presenting with complaints of hearing loss, disequilibrium, vertigo, or a combination of these symptoms. Ménière disease, vestibular migraine, labyrinthitis or vestibular neuritis, autoimmune hearing loss, otosyphilis, and classic vestibular schwannomas of the IAC or CPA are all considered. Typically, the clinician has to decide between possible diagnoses based on the appearance of an enhancing inner ear lesion seen on an MRI. This list can generally be divided into primary enhancing lesions confined to the inner ear or enhancing lesions that extend to and include the inner ear. Labyrinthine hemorrhage (**Fig. 5**) is a relatively rare diagnosis, which presents similar to acute viral labyrinthitis (**Fig. 6**) in patients with concussive head trauma or spontaneously in patients on anticoagulant therapy. Chronic labyrinthitis with or without ossification is a cause of SNHL secondary to bacterial meningitis in children and adults (**Fig. 7**). All of these MRI abnormalities show a more diffuse inner ear enhancement without discrete borders. Alternatively, ILS presents as a discrete enhancement with sharply marginated borders on both contrast-enhanced T1-weighted and CISS T2-weighted sequences (**Fig. 8**).

There are several very rare case reports of primary tumors arising within the labyrinth. One such case reported a recurrent (or residual) cochlear ILS after resection of an IAC vestibular schwannoma.[34] A few intralabyrinthine lipomas have been reported, and these were diagnosed by suppression of tumor hyperintensity on fat-suppression T1-weighted MRI sequences.[35] Another case report highlighted a traumatic neuroma following labyrinthectomy.[36] This patient had a remote history of Ménière disease treated with labyrinthectomy and then later developed a more chronic dysequilibrium.[4] However, it is not entirely certain if the traumatic neuroma was truly causative of the imbalance. Lastly, the senior authors have treated a patient who presented with unilateral deafness and an MRI showing a discrete inner ear lesion similar to an ILS. However, the tumor showed atypical T1 hyperintensity without contrast and an extremely rapid growth rate to involve the CPA. Surgical pathology confirmed the diagnosis of melanocytic schwannoma arising from the vestibule (**Fig. 9**).

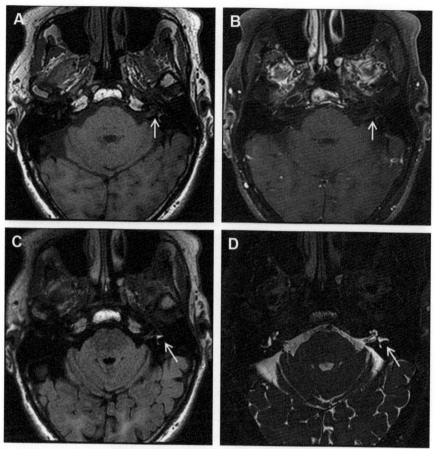

Fig. 5. Acute hemorrhage in left vestibule. (*A*) Axial precontrast 3D fast spin echo T1-weighted image shows mild T1 hyperintensity (*arrow*) consistent with hemorrhage; (*B*) axial postcontrast T1-weighted image (*arrow*) does not exhibit any contrast enhancement; (*C*) axial 3D fluid-attenuated inversion recovery image demonstrates subtle hyperintense signal within the vestibule and adjacent semicircular canal (*arrow*) consistent with hemorrhage; (*D*) axial 3D fast spin echo T2-weighted image shows normal labyrinthine fluid signal intensity, which can often mask signal from intralabyrinthine hemorrhage (*arrow*).

There are also rare instances when tumors or inflammatory lesions arise outside the inner ear but extend to involve the cochlea or vestibule. Meningiomas of the IAC (**Fig. 10**), lymphoma (**Fig. 11**), posttransplant lymphoproliferative disease (PTLD) (**Fig. 12**), and paraganglioma (**Fig. 13**) can all present with unilateral SNHL and vestibular complaints. The MRI appearance can be similar to an ILS that has extended to involve the IAC or middle ear.

MANAGEMENT AND OUTCOMES
Management

The treatment approach for ILS is dictated by patient symptoms, tumor size, and tumor location. Surgical indications for ILS removal are intractable vertigo, growth into the IAC or middle ear, and uncertainty regarding diagnosis.[1,4,6,7,18] Management

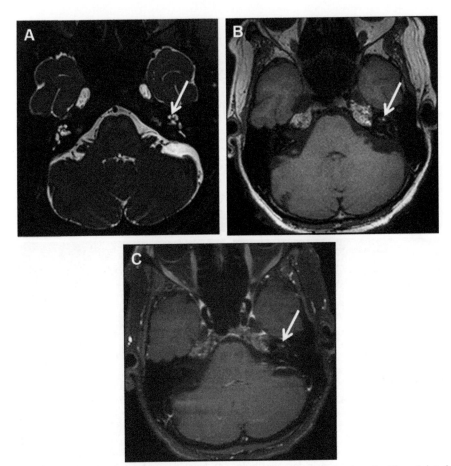

Fig. 6. Acute labyrinthitis with hemorrhage, left ear. (*A*) Axial 3D fast spin echo T2-weighted image shows normal fluid signal within the inner ear and cochlea (*arrow*); (*B*) axial precontrast 3D fast spine echo T1-weighted image shows signal hyperintensity of the cochlea (*arrow*); (*C*) axial fat-saturated postcontrast 3D fast spin echo T1-weighted image demonstrates no substantial enhancement (*arrow*).

options primarily include observation with serial MRI versus surgical removal, with the approach dictated by tumor size and location. To the authors' knowledge, only 2 patients have been reported that received stereotactic radiosurgery (SRS) for their ILS.[1,6] There has also been a single report using transtympanic steroid injections for a patient with ILS with sudden SNHL.[37] This patient experienced short-term hearing improvement until the inevitable tumor induced SNHL.

In a 2013 ILS review, 53% of patients (109 of 189) were observed with serial MRI scans. Only 3% of observed patients went on to need surgical removal because of vestibular symptoms or significant tumor growth. This finding was despite MRI evidence of slow tumor growth in 52% of these patients. They found that in the observation group, 93% (55 of 59) had stable or improved tinnitus, unsteadiness, or vertigo.[6] These findings provide support for a more conservative approach to the management of these tumors.

When patients experience severe vertigo or tumor growth into the IAC, CPA, or middle ear, treatment is required. Earlier removal of these tumors before extensive

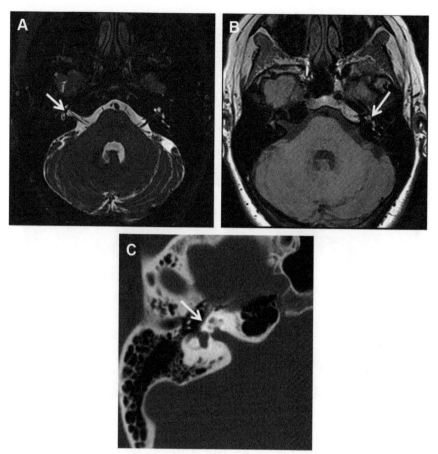

Fig. 7. Bilateral autoimmune labyrinthitis with ossification on the right and hemorrhage on the left. (A) Axial 3D fast spin echo T2-weighted image demonstrates loss of fluid in the right cochlea (*arrow*) consistent with chronic labyrinthitis; (B) axial precontrast 3D fast spin echo T1-weighted image shows T1 hyperintensity of the labyrinth indicating hemorrhage (*arrow*) secondary to subacute labyrinthitis; (C) axial CT shows cochlear ossification (*arrow*) correlating with the loss of fluid signal as demonstrated in (A).

IAC involvement is likely to have less risk of postoperative facial paralysis.[38] Middle ear ILS extension has also historically been an indication for tumor removal. The provided reasoning for this is that the tumor lacks a barrier to spread once it has reached the middle ear. This decision is probably sound in more quickly growing tumors, but it can be questioned in most slow-growing tumors. The middle ear may provide slow-growing tumors an increased area to asymptomatically expand without consequence. In general, the senior author removes tumors with middle ear extension through the oval window because of the proximity of the tympanic facial nerve. This practice allows tumor removal when facial nerve contact is at a minimum and may provide easier dissection and facial nerve preservation. Additionally, middle ear ILS are also removed before significant eustachian tube involvement because this can add a degree of difficulty to complete tumor resection. Slow-growing tumors extending through the round window into the hypotympanum might be observed if they have not radiographically encroached on the facial nerve.

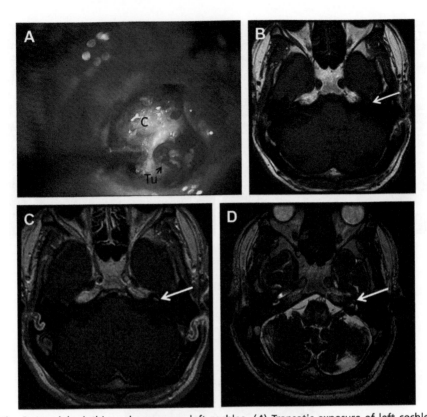

Fig. 8. Intralabyrinthine schwannoma, left cochlea. (*A*) Transotic exposure of left cochlea schwannoma; (*B*) axial precontrast T1-weighted image shows normal T1 hypointensity signal within left cochlea (*arrow*); (*C*) axial postcontrast T1-weighted image demonstrates enhancement of the basal turn of the cochlea (*arrow*); (*D*) axial 3D gradient echo T2-weighted image shows filling defect (hypointensity) within the bright cochlear fluid signal (*arrow*). C, petrous internal carotid artery; Tu, tumor within the basal turn of cochlea.

Clinicians may rarely be faced with a patient with ILS experiencing severe vertigo without tumor growth or hearing loss. Transtympanic gentamicin injection could be done in these instances especially if that patient did not wish to have surgery or was medically unfit for surgery. Patients should be counseled that this treatment does not prevent tumor growth and any remaining hearing could be lost because of the injection.

Ultimately, most patients requiring treatment will undergo surgical removal. It is helpful to have ILS classification schemes in order to choose an appropriate surgical approach for the tumor location. It is important that patients understand that they will no longer have any hearing regardless of the surgical approach selected, although most patients with these ILS present with nonserviceable hearing.[6] Patients with tumors isolated to the vestibular system (vestibule or semicircular canals) can effectively undergo tumor removal via a transmastoid labyrinthectomy. If there is extension of a labyrinth ILS into the IAC or CPA, the translabyrinthine approach provides adequate exposure for tumor resection. Patients with cochlear involvement are likely to require a transotic approach for ILS removal, regardless of whether there is tumor extension into the IAC. This approach would also provide adequate exposure for cochlear tumors involving the middle ear (see **Fig. 8**). The transotic approach requires overclosure of the external auditory meatus, packing of the middle ear, and eustachian

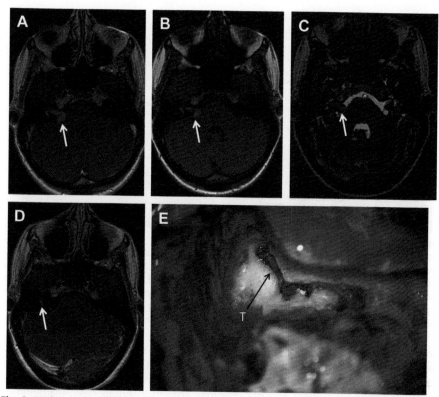

Fig. 9. Melanocytic schwannoma, right ear. (*A*) Axial precontrast T1-weighted image shows a tumor involving the vestibule, internal auditory canal, and CPA (*arrow*). The tumor is T1 hyperintense despite the absence of contrast, which is not typical of an ILS or vestibular schwannoma; (*B*) axial postcontrast T1-weighted image shows slight increase in tumor enhancement compared with the T1 precontrast image (*arrow*); (*C*) axial 3D gradient echo T2-weighted image demonstrates a corresponding fluid void (hypointensity) in the area of the tumor (*arrow*); (*D*) axial T1 contrast-enhanced MRI from 2 years before the MRI in (*A–C*). There is an enhancing lesion involving only the vestibule (*arrow*). This lesion was initially interpreted as an ILS; however, the same precontrast T1 hyperintensity was also present within the vestibule. This atypical enhancement and rapid growth are not seen with ILS; (*E*) Right translabyrinthine exposure of tumor (T) filling the vestibule. Note the marked black pigmentation of the tumor; histopathology diagnosed a melanocytic schwannoma.

tube obliteration to prevent CSF leak from the IAC through the basal cochlear modiolus. Tumors with only minimal cochlear involvement could potentially be removed without a transotic approach. Case reports of transmastoid removal of small cochlear, basal turn ILS have been published. The authors describe a standard facial recess approach and enlarged cochleostomy for tumor removal.[39] Additionally, older reports exist of transcanal removal of ILS found unexpectedly in patients undergoing transcanal labyrinthectomy.[4] However, this is probably not advisable as a planned procedure because vestibule tumor exposure and removal might be incomplete.

Outcomes

To date, no operated patient has developed tumor recurrence after gross total ILS excision, but long-term imaging follow-up was not available for many case series.

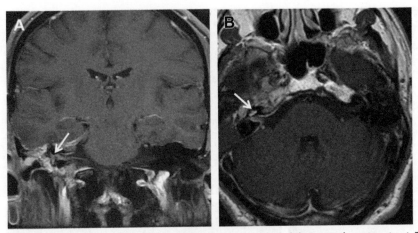

Fig. 10. Meningioma involving the right IAC and cochlea. (*A*) Coronal postcontrast T1-weighted image shows abnormal enhancement of the vestibule (*arrow*) and visualized semicircular canals, with extension into the adjacent IAC, particularly along the superior dural surface; (*B*) axial postcontrast T1-weighted image shows abnormal enhancement of the cochlea (*arrow*) and dural lining of the IAC, extending to involve the dura overlying the adjacent CPA. The dural tail enhancement is most typical of a meningioma. This dural thickening is more often a reactive process rather than direct tumor invasion of the dura.

One patient, who underwent subtotal tumor removal, required a second surgery because of residual tumor growth in the cochlea after an initial transotic approach.[40] Surgical excision of ILS has resulted in vertigo resolution in many patients, although patient selection for surgery was not uniformly applied.[1,7] Additionally, utilization of standardized vestibular symptom definitions was also not performed. It is unlikely that spontaneous-onset vertigo was systematically distinguished from head-motion induced vertigo, disequilibrium while walking, or constant dizziness present in all positions and activities.

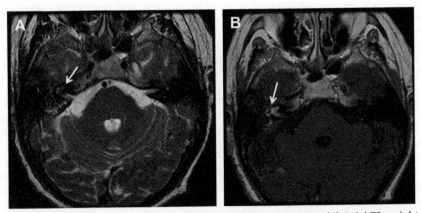

Fig. 11. B-cell lymphoma of the distal right IAC and entire inner ear. (*A*) Axial T2-weighted image shows absence of normal fluid in the right cochlea (*arrow*) and distal IAC, with T2-hypointense material; (*B*) axial postcontrast T1-weighted image shows homogenous enhancement of this same tissue (*arrow*). Lymphoma is often T2 hypointense because of its high nuclear/cytoplasmic ratio and usually demonstrates homogenous enhancement.

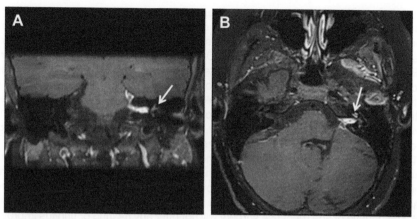

Fig. 12. PTLD seen in the left IAC, CPA, and inner ear. (*A*) Coronal reformatted fat-suppressed postcontrast 3D fast spin echo T1-weighted image shows prominent enhancement throughout the left IAC, extending along the proximal cistern superiorly, with faint enhancement of the adjacent left semicircular canals (*arrow*); (*B*) axial fat suppressed postcontrast 3D fast spin echo T1-weighted image shows the prominent enhancement of the left IAC and adjacent posterior cistern, with enhancement of the left cochlea (*arrow*).

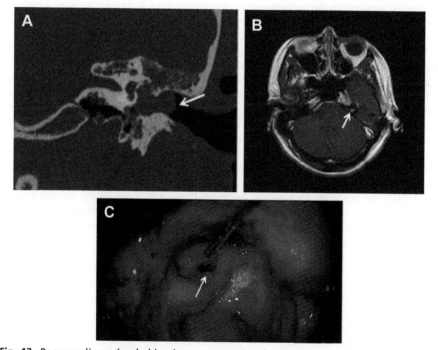

Fig. 13. Paraganglioma (probable glomus tympanicum) originating in the left middle ear. Extension to involve the left external auditory canal, vestibule, and distal IAC is shown. (*A*) Coronal CT image shows soft tissue filling the medial left external auditory canal (*arrow*) with opacification of the adjacent mastoid air cells and mild demineralization; (*B*) axial postcontrast T1-weighted image shows an small enhancing mass in the visualized left IAC (*arrow*); (*C*) surgical view of the left ear in which the canal wall has been removed. The basal turn of the cochlea has been opened with paraganglioma tumor found filling the lumen (*arrow*).

Complications after ILS surgery are seemingly rare. Unfortunately, facial nerve outcomes are difficult to assess because of the sporadic reporting practices in the literature. Postoperative facial nerve paresis or paralysis was an unusual complication seen in 4% (2 of 55) of surgical patients. One patient initially had House-Brackmann (HB) grade III/VI facial paresis that completely resolved by 1 year, and another patient had HB grade IV function 12 months postoperatively.[1,7] There have been 3 cases of patients experiencing postsurgical CSF leak.[25,26] One of these was managed conservatively, whereas one required a second operation on the development of meningitis. Two of these were managed conservatively, whereas one required a second operation to control the CSF leak after the development of meningitis.

There are a few controversies regarding the management of ILS. The first is regarding whether young patients (≤50 years old) with a slowly growing ILS should undergo prolonged observation, even if they lack vestibular symptoms. As previously highlighted, many surgeons promote a wait-and-scan policy in all patients with nonvertiginous ILS, irrespective of age, because surgery will not offer any hearing or tinnitus improvement. On the other hand, even if growth is limited to 1 mm every 2 to 3 years, the tumor will likely run out of room within the inner ear and extend to the IAC at some point over the next 30 to 40 years. This transmodiolar or transmacular ILS would then need treatment in a more elderly patient group. Of course treatment could be accomplished with stereotactic radiotherapy; but because of this probable need to treat within a patients' lifetime, surgery should probably be a treatment option discussed with younger (≤50 years-old), asymptomatic patients with a slowly growing ILS. Moreover, even with conservative MRI follow-up schedules every 2 to 5 years, this is a large commitment of patient time and medical resources over younger patients' lifetime.

The second controversy surrounding ILS management is whether SRS should be considered a valid, first-line treatment option. There have been 2 reports of SRS treatment of ILS. One of these patients that underwent SRS had no clinical or radiographic follow-up.[1] The second patient underwent successful SRS following tumor growth on serial MRI scans.[6] Hearing preservation is probably not possible due to the high cochlear radiation dose, and SRS treatment should not be considered until AAO-HNS class D hearing levels are reached. The indications for SRS could potentially be similar for ILS and IAC schwannomas; this would include tumor growth on serial MRI scans, growth of the tumor to involve the IAC, and intractable spontaneous vertigo. Imbalance, constant dizziness, and motion-provoked vertigo are not good SRS (or surgical) indications because these are more likely resultant from poor central compensation rather than an irritative tumor phenomena. There is some hesitancy to recommend SRS to treat ILS tumors causing spontaneous vertigo because, theoretically, the tumor that is causing abnormal vestibular input has not been removed. Surgical removal of ILS tumors also accomplishes total vestibular ablation, which may allow patients better spontaneous vertigo control. These hypotheses have not really been well studied in the treatment of ILS or standard vestibular schwannomas. Lastly, the risk-benefit analysis for ILS tumors is different from standard IAC or CPA tumors. Complete microsurgical removal of ILS tumors without IAC involvement is generally easily accomplished, and the risk of facial nerve morbidity is limited compared with standard vestibular schwannomas. Currently, SRS for the treatment of ILS has been reserved for the medically infirm who cannot undergo surgical anesthesia. With the relative infrequency of these tumors, the slow growth, and the difficulty in measuring growth on serial scans, it is unlikely that a randomized, prospective trial comparing SRS, microsurgery, and observation will ever occur. Future outcomes research will be needed to assist in defining best treatment practices.

HEARING REHABILITATION

Increasingly, patients with unilateral, profound SNHL are finding significant benefit from cochlear implantation (CI). CI restores a degree of bilateral hearing that may help with sound localization and hearing in noise that cannot be provided by contralateral routing of sound strategies.[41] Currently, in the United States, insurance companies do not provide reimbursement for CI when the contralateral ear has normal or near-normal hearing. Although speculative, the authors postulate that eventually CI for unilateral hearing loss will become more mainstream with consistent outcome studies to demonstrate a benefit. The use of CI in unilateral deafness is significant for patients with ILS because most of these patients will have unilateral, profound SNHL in need of rehabilitation. CI rehabilitation might also shift the current ILS treatment paradigm away from observation to early surgical removal at a time when the tumor is at its smallest. Obviously there are many unanswered questions as to whether this will be possible for patients with ILS. Most likely, patients with tumors limited to the vestibule and semicircular canals will be able to undergo simultaneous tumor removal and successful CI with resultant hearing benefit. Alternatively, cochlear ILS may be difficult to remove while still maintaining enough cochlear spiral ganglion cells and distal cochlear nerve branches to ensure significant CI benefit. Two cases of resection of limited cochlear schwannomas from the basal turn have been reported with simultaneous CI placement.[39,42] Initial hearing results were good in one patient, although long-term follow-up and standardized sentence testing comparison with patients with typical CI was not performed. It is also not clear if CI would need to be performed at primary tumor extirpation or whether it could be done in a delayed fashion. If CI placement were staged over concerns of CSF leakage, the window of time for successful CI insertion is also not established. Worry over delayed labyrinthitis ossificans development, and subsequent implantation failure, has been highlighted in case studies of patients who previously underwent labyrinthectomy.[43] However, how quickly this develops and in what percentage of patients is currently not clear.

SUMMARY

ILS are uncommon tumors that were historically found either at the time of autopsy or unexpectedly during surgery for control of vertigo in patients thought to have Ménière disease. Numerous retrospective case reports, case series, and literature reviews have increased our knowledge of these tumors. The routine use of high-resolution MRI has increased the likelihood of discovering these tumors and has subsequently increased their incidence. Armed with the knowledge of their clinical presentation and overlap with other neurotologic pathology, as well as the imaging specifics required to visualize these tumors, clinicians will certainly decrease delays in diagnosis. Although a conservative wait-and-scan approach can be used for most patients, operative management is often indicated and results in rare morbidity. Future reports may help in both expanding surgical indications and further clarifying if there is a role for primary SRS.

REFERENCES

1. Kennedy RJ, Shelton C, Salzman KL, et al. Intralabyrinthine schwannomas: diagnosis, management, and a new classification system. Otol Neurotol 2004;25: 160–7.
2. Driscoll CL. Vestibular schwannoma. In: Driscoll CL, editor. Tumors of the ear and temporal bone. Philadelphia: Lippincott Williams & Wilkins; 2000. p. 172–218.

3. Jackler RT, Brackmann DE. Acoustic neuroma (vestibular schwannoma). In: Jackler RT, editor. Neurotology. Philadelphia: Mosby, Inc; 2005. p. 727–82.
4. Green J. Intralabyrinthine schwannoma. In: Driscoll CL, editor. Tumors of the ear and temporal bone. Philadelphia: Lippincott Williams & Wilkins; 2000. p. 146–55.
5. Mayer O. Ein Fall von multiplen Tumoren in den Endansbreitungen des Akustikus. Z Ohrenheilk 1917;75:95–113.
6. Van Abel KV, Carlson ML, Link MJ, et al. Primary inner ear schwannomas: a case series and systematic review of the literature. Laryngoscope 2013;123(8):1957–66.
7. Neff BA, Willcox TO, Sataloff RT. Intralabyrinthine schwannomas. Otol Neurotol 2003;24:299–307.
8. Anson BJ, Donaldson JA, editors. Surgical anatomy of the temporal bone. Philadelphia: WB Saunders; 1981. p. 475–81.
9. Donnelly M, Daly C, Briggs R. MR imaging features of an intracochlear acoustic schwannoma. J Laryngol Otol 1994;108:1111–4.
10. O'Keefe LJ, Camilleri AE, Gillespie JE, et al. Primary tumors of the vestibule and inner ear. J Laryngol Otol 1997;111:709–14.
11. Sterkers JM, Perre J, Viola P, et al. The origin of acoustic neuromas. Acta Otolaryngol 1987;103:427–31.
12. Xenellis JE, Linthicum FH. On the myth of glial/Schwann junction (Obersteiner-Redlich zone): origin of vestibular nerve schwannomas. Otol Neurotol 2003;24:1.
13. Gussen R. Intramodular acoustic neurilemoma. Laryngoscope 1971;81:1979–84.
14. Babin RW, Harker LA. Intralabyrinthine acoustic neuromas. Otolaryngol Head Neck Surg 1980;88:455–61.
15. Jorgensen MB. Intracochlear neuroma. Acta Otolaryngol 1960;54:227–32.
16. Johnson LG, Kingsley TC. Asymptomatic intracochlear neuroma. A temporal bone report. Arch Otolaryngol 1981;107:377–81.
17. Amoils CP, Lanser MJ, Jackler RK. Acoustic neuroma presenting as a middle ear mass. Otolaryngol Head Neck Surg 1992;107:478–82.
18. Stoney PJ, Rurka J, Dolan E, et al. Acoustic neuroma presenting as a middle ear mass. J Otolaryngol 1991;20:141–3.
19. Doyle KJ, Brackmann DE. Intralabyrinthine schwannomas. Otolaryngol Head Neck Surg 1994;110:517–23.
20. Committee on Hearing and Equilibrium guidelines for the evaluation of hearing preservation in acoustic neuroma (vestibular schwannoma). American Academy of Otolaryngology–Head and Neck Surgery Foundation, INC. Otolaryngol Head Neck Surg 1995;113:179–80.
21. DeLozier HL, Gacek RR, Dana ST. Intralabyrinthine schwannoma. Ann Otol Rhinol Laryngol 1979;88:187–91.
22. Miyamoto RT, Isenberg SF, Culp WM, et al. Isolated intralabyrinthine schwannoma. Am J Otol 1980;1:215–7.
23. Hallpike CS. Stapes fixation by an intralabyrinthine 'seedling' neurofibroma as a cause of conductive deafness in a case of von Recklinghausen's disease. Acta Otolaryngol Suppl 1963;183:62–5.
24. Hamed A, Linthicum F. Intralabyrinthine Schwannoma. Otol Neurotol 2005;26:1085–6.
25. Storrs LA. Acoustic neuromas presenting as middle ear tumors. Laryngoscope 1974;84:1175–80.
26. Tran Ba Huy P, Hassan JM, Wassef M, et al. Acoustic schwannoma presenting as a tumor of the external auditory canal. Ann Otol Rhinol Laryngol 1987;96:415–7.
27. Karlan MS, Besek M, Potter GB. Intracochlear neurilemoma. Arch Otolaryngol 1972;96:573–5.

28. Wanamaker HH. Acoustic neuroma primary arising in the vestibule. Laryngoscope 1972;82:1040–4.
29. Vernick DM, Graham MD, McClatchey KD. Intralabyrinthine schwannoma. Laryngoscope 1984;94:1241–3.
30. Hawke M, Keene M, Robbins KT, et al. Occult labyrinthine schwannoma. J Otolaryngol 1981;10:313–20.
31. Mafee M, Lachenauer CS, Kamar A, et al. CT and MR imaging of intralabyrinthine schwannoma: report of two cases and review of the literature. Radiology 1990; 174:395–400.
32. Lane JI, Witte RJ, Bolster B, et al. State of the art: 3T imaging of the membranous labyrinth. AJNR Am J Neuroradiol 2008;29:1436–40.
33. Casselman JW, Kuhweide R, Deimling M, et al. Constructive interference in steady state-3DFT-MR imaging of the inner ear and cerebellopontine angle. AJNR Am J Neuroradiol 1993;14:47–57.
34. Green JD Jr, Beatty CW, Czervionke LF, et al. Intracochlear vestibular schwannoma: a potential source for recurrence after translabyrinthine resection. Otolaryngol Head Neck Surg 2000;123:281–2.
35. Dahlen RT, Johnson CE, Harnsberger HR, et al. CT and MR imaging characteristics of intravestibular lipoma. AJNR Am J Neuroradiol 2002;23(8):1413–7.
36. Linthicum FH, Alonso A, Denia A. Traumatic neuroma: a complication of transcanal labyrinthectomy. Arch Otolaryngol 1979;105:654–5.
37. Iseri M, Ulubil SA, Topdag M, et al. Hearing loss owing to intralabyrinthine schwannoma responsive to intratympanic steroid treatment. J Otolaryngol Head Neck Surg 2009;38:E95–7.
38. Moffat DA, Parker PA, Hardy DG, et al. Factors affecting final facial nerve outcome following vestibular schwannoma surgery. J Laryngol Otol 2014; 128(5):406–15.
39. Schutt CA, Kveton JF. Cochlear implantation after resection of an intralabyrinthine schwannoma. Am J Otolaryngol 2014;35:257–60.
40. Falcioni M, Taibah A, DiTrapani G, et al. Inner ear extension of vestibular schwannomas. Laryngoscope 2003;113:1605–8.
41. Blasco MA, Redleaf MI. Cochlear implantation in unilateral sudden deafness improves tinnitus and speech comprehension: meta-analysis and systematic review. Otol Neurotol 2014;35(8):1426–32.
42. Kronenberg J, Horowitz Z, Hildesheimer M. Intracochlear schwannoma and cochlear implantation. Ann Otol Rhinol Laryngol 1999;108:659–60.
43. Chen DA, Linthicum FH Jr, Rizer FM. Cochlear histopathology in the labyrinthectomized ear: implications for cochlear implantation. Laryngoscope 1988;98(11): 1170–2.

Neurofibromatosis Type 2

William H. Slattery, MD

KEYWORDS

- Neurofibromatosis type 2 • Vestibular schwannoma • Acoustic neuroma

KEY POINTS

- Care of patients with neurofibromatosis type 2 (NF2) requires knowledge of all tumors and symptoms involved with the disorder.
- It is recommended that patients receive care in a center with expertise in NF2.
- The role of the neuro-otologist in this care is determined by the specialty center.

INTRODUCTION

Neurofibromatosis (NF) is a rare syndrome characterized by bilateral vestibular schwannomas, multiple meningiomas, cranial nerve (CN) tumors, spinal tumors, and eye abnormalities. Neurofibromatosis type 2 (NF2) presents unique challenges to the otologist because hearing loss may be the presenting complaint leading to the diagnosis of the disorder. NF2 is invasive, requiring a multispecialist team approach for the evaluation and treatment of the disorder. The primary impairment is hearing loss resulting from bilateral vestibular schwannomas. NF2 must be differentiated from neurofibromatosis type 1 (NF1); although the names are linked, the disease entities are distinctly different. This article reviews the clinical characteristics of NF2 and current recommendations for evaluation and treatment.

NEUROFIBROMATOSIS TYPE 2 DIFFERENTIATED FROM NEUROFIBROMATOSIS TYPE 1

NF1 has distinctly different characteristics from NF2. NF1 and NF2 have been distinguished as completely different genetic diseases based on the chromosome responsible for the disease. NF1 has been localized to chromosome 17, and NF2 has been localized to chromosome 22. NF1 is a multisystem disorder in which some features may be present at birth and others are age-related manifestations. The National Institutes of Health (NIH) Consensus Development Conference identified the following 7

Disclosure: No funding or other support was required for this study.
Conflict of Interest: The authors report no conflicts of interest concerning the information presented in this article.
House Clinic, 2100 West 3rd Street, Suite 111, Los Angeles, CA 90057, USA
E-mail address: wslattery@hei.org

Otolaryngol Clin N Am 48 (2015) 443–460
http://dx.doi.org/10.1016/j.otc.2015.02.005
0030-6665/15/$ – see front matter © 2015 Elsevier Inc. All rights reserved.

oto.theclinics.com

features of the disease, of which 2 or more are required to establish the diagnosis of NF1:

1. Six café au lait spots equal to or greater than 5 mm in longest diameter in prepubertal patients and 15 mm in longest diameter in postpubertal patients
2. Two or more neurofibromas of any type or 1 plexiform neurofibroma
3. Freckling in the axilla or inguinal regions
4. Optic glioma (optic pathway glioma)
5. Two or more Lisch nodules (iris, hamartoma)
6. Distinct osseous lesions, such as sphenoid wing dysplasia or cortical thinning of the cortex of long bones with or without pseudoarthrosis
7. First-degree relative (parent, sibling, or child) with NF1 according to the criteria listed earlier

Some patients also manifest learning disabilities or language disorders. A careful examination and a detailed history of the patient's symptoms help distinguish NF1 and NF2.

CLINICAL CHARACTERISTICS OF NEUROFIBROMATOSIS TYPE 2
Definition

The NIH Consensus Development Conference also developed guidelines for the diagnosis of NF2. NF2 is distinguished by bilateral vestibular schwannomas with multiple meningiomas, CN tumors, optic gliomas, and spinal tumors. A definite diagnosis is made from the presence of bilateral vestibular schwannomas or developing a unilateral vestibular schwannoma by age 30 years and a first-degree blood relative with NF2, or the presence of a unilateral vestibular schwannoma and developing at least 2 of the following conditions known to be associated with NF2: meningioma, glioma, schwannoma, or juvenile posterior subcapsular lenticular opacity/juvenile cortical cataract (**Box 1**).[1]

Box 1
NF2 diagnostic criteria

Confirmed (definite) NF2

Bilateral VS or family history of NF2 (first-degree family relative) plus

1. Unilateral VS less than 30 years, or

2. Any 2 of the following: meningioma, glioma, schwannoma, juvenile posterior subcapsular lenticular opacities/juvenile cortical cataract

Presumptive or probable NF2: should evaluate for NF2

Unilateral VS less than 30 years plus at least 1 of the following:

    Meningioma, glioma, schwannoma, juvenile posterior subcapsular lenticular opacities/juvenile cortical cataract

Multiple meningiomas (≥2) plus unilateral VS less than 30 years or one of the following:

    Glioma, schwannoma, juvenile posterior subcapsular lenticular opacities/juvenile cortical cataract

Abbreviation: VS, vestibular schwannoma.

Adapted from Slattery WH. Neurofibromatosis 2 in otologic surgery. In: Brackmann DE, Shelton C, Arriaga MA, editors. Philadelphia: Elsevier; 2010. p. 691–701; with permission.

There may be significant heterogeneity in the presentation of the disease from one individual to the next. Some individuals may have a very mild form of the disease, such as small vestibular schwannomas manifesting in an older individual. At the other end of the spectrum, some children present with multiple intracranial tumors at a very young age. Despite the heterogeneity of the disease, the expression of NF2 tends to be similar within a family.[2] There is a significant genetic component to the disease with much variability within the parameters of the observed phenotype. Studies have shown that a truncating mutation (nonsense and frame shift) may be linked to a more severe form of NF2.[3,4] The more severe form of NF2 is termed the Wishart form. Individuals with this severe form present with early onset of the disease, with multiple intracranial schwannomas and meningiomas that result in blindness, deafness, paralysis, and possibly death by age 40 years. Despite the strong genotype-phenotype correlation seen in NF2, individual differences in tumor growth occur within patients, making it difficult to predict how an individual's tumors will change over time even when the genotype is known. The milder form, the Gardner form, of NF2 is less debilitating. Schwannomas may remain stable for many years, few meningiomas develop, and patients may not develop symptoms until later in life and often have fewer associated disabilities. The genetic basis of the mild form has not been well characterized. Many of these may be mosaic forms of the disease.[2-10]

Prevalence and Incidence

The average age of diagnosis of NF2 is 25 years; however, many patients present with symptoms before the diagnosis. There is an average delay of diagnosis of approximately 7 years.[11] There is no difference in the proportion of men versus women who develop NF2, and no prevalence has been described based on ethnicity. Epidemiologic studies place the incidence of NF2 between 1 in 33,000 live births[3] and 1 in 87,410 live births.[12]

Imaging Studies

All patients suspected to have NF2 should have a high-quality MRI scan performed with thin cuts through the internal auditory canals (IAC). All patients diagnosed with a unilateral vestibular schwannoma should have a dedicated IAC series to ensure there is not another tumor on the opposite side. Patients diagnosed with NF2 should have a complete spine series to evaluate the spine and stage the disease. Small spinal tumors commonly may be found in the cauda equina area, and occasionally a large asymptomatic schwannoma or meningioma may be found in the spine that could require treatment. Early treatment of spine tumors can significantly reduce the morbidity associated with these lesions. It is unusual for patients older than 40 years to present with NF2, although with more sensitive MRI scanning techniques, more of these individuals are being diagnosed at an older age. Metastasis may rarely manifest with bilateral IAC lesions, and it is important that carcinoma be ruled out in any patient older than 40 years who presents with bilateral IAC lesions.

A patient identified with NF2 should have a complete cranial MRI scan with cervical thoracic and lumbar spinal imaging. This scan serves as a baseline. A 6-month follow-up MRI scan is recommended for the intracranial tumors. If the tumors show stability, a yearly MRI scan is performed on the intracranial structures. Large tumors in the spine may be monitored with a similar frequency. If no spinal tumors are present, spinal imaging should be performed if the patient becomes symptomatic. Monitoring spinal tumors every 3 years is recommended when these are present. Intracranial imaging is performed on a yearly basis unless studies over several years indicate stability of the tumors.

Molecular Genetics

The NF2 gene was mapped to chromosome 22q12–2 in 1993.[13–15] The NF2 gene located at chromosome 22 codes for a tumor suppressive protein termed merlin or schwannomin. This protein negatively regulates Schwann cell production and the loss of this protein allows overproduction of Schwann cells. The mutation in the NF2 chain predisposes individuals to developing a schwannoma when the second hit occurs to the gene; control of Schwann cells is lost or mutated within the cell. Various types of mutations have been identified, including single-base substitutions, insertions, and deletions.[2,4,16–18] The mild, or Gardner, type of NF2 may be associated with missense mutations, whereas associations between the other mutations and phenotypes are not as clear.[10] The occurrence of NF2 is not restricted to families known to carry the mutation. Frequently, genetic mosaicism occurs, which may not be detected by common mutation analysis techniques.[19] Unilateral vestibular schwannomas may show the same type of genetic markers as NF2.[20] The mutations in unilateral vestibular schwannomas are confined to the affected tumor tissue. In patients with NF2, the mutation is present in all cell types.[19]

Family History

NF2 is an autosomal dominant disease, and 50% of children of affected individuals are at risk for developing the disease. Of patients in whom NF2 is diagnosed, 50% present with a family history of NF2. Half of all NF2-affected patients have no family history of NF2 and are considered founder cases. NF2 presentation and phenotype tend to be similar within families. The likelihood of NF2 occurring in related individuals who do not show similar clinical symptoms to an affected family member is small. Consideration must still be given to screening these individuals for risks despite the lack of clinical symptoms. Individuals at risk for developing NF2 must be screened to provide an early diagnosis. Individuals at risk include children of NF2-affected patients and their siblings. Fifty percent of all children of patients with NF2 are found to have the disease. Siblings of a patient diagnosed with NF1 are at risk, especially if the parent also has NF2. The type of screening and timing of screening depend on each NF2 center's preference. Early screening is advocated so that tumors may be diagnosed presymptomatically. Screening may occur via MRI or genetic blood testing.

Screening

MRI screening of potentially affected individuals uses a postcontrast T1-weighted sequence of the full head with thin cuts through the IAC. A dedicated IAC MRI scan identifies most patients with NF2 by showing any vestibular schwannomas. Screening of the spine and ophthalmologic examination should be considered if the cranial MRI scan is positive. An audiogram (pure tone thresholds) or current clinical standard auditory brainstem response (ABR) testing is likely to miss small vestibular schwannomas. MRI can diagnose presymptomatically.

MRI is recommended for at-risk children when this test can be performed without sedation; this usually can be done when the child is 7 to 9 years old. A recommended first step for children younger than 7 years is an audiogram. Any child with an NF2-associated symptom, such as hearing loss or facial weakness, should be screened without regard to the need for sedation or age; MRI should be performed as soon as possible after the symptoms become apparent.

Identification of the NF2 gene and chromosome 22 has made genetic testing possible. It is recommended that patients with NF2 see a genetic counselor to discuss the hereditary consequences of the disease. Blood testing for the mutation is able to identify the defect of the NF2 gene in approximately 70% to 75% of patients with a known diagnosis of NF2. If the defect is identified in the affected individual, potential family members may be screened. If the gene is not identified in the affected individuals, blood screening of family members cannot be performed. The use of blood screening for patients without a diagnosis of NF2 or with a suspected diagnosis of NF2 is not recommended. New mutations in patients with mild presentation are most likely to be missense mutations, and this is difficult to identify with genetic testing of patients with NF2. The best molecular testing is performed on fresh vestibular schwannoma tissue. Any patient with a planned vestibular schwannoma removal should be offered the opportunity to have their tumor tissue tested for the genetic mutation. This test is the most sensitive and allows identification of the genetic mutation in most cases. The results of this test can then be used to screen relatives for NF2. There are currently 2 clinical laboratories that perform this test (Massachusetts General and University of Alabama) and there are many research laboratories associated with NF centers that may perform the test on recently resected tissue. The tissue must be keep frozen and testing should be coordinated with the laboratories before surgical resection.

SCHWANNOMA TUMOR TYPES

Bilateral vestibular schwannomas (acoustic neuromas) are benign neoplasms of the acoustic or eighth CN (**Fig. 1**).[21] The tumors are thought to arise at the glioma–Schwann cell junction within the internal auditory meatus. The tumors most commonly arise from the superior vestibular nerve, although, with NF2, tumors may be found on the cochlear and facial nerves within the internal auditory meatus. The consequences

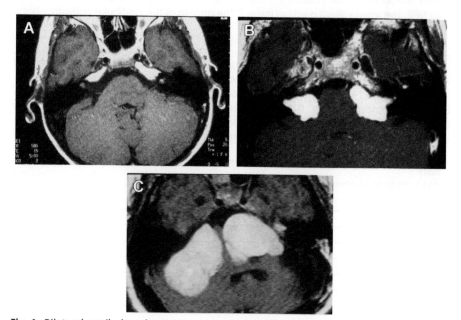

Fig. 1. Bilateral vestibular schwannomas are characteristic of NF2. (*A*) Small bilateral vestibular schwannomas. (*B*) Medium-sized vestibular schwannomas that are compressing the brainstem. (*C*) Giant bilateral vestibular schwannomas that are compressing the brainstem and causing hydrocephalus.

of a vestibular schwannoma are numerous, including hearing loss progressing to deafness; dizziness and balance problems; tinnitus; facial nerve paralysis; brainstem compression; and, if left untreated, death.

Despite the strong genetic effect in NF2, there is enormous variability in the number of tumor types, the rate of progression, and the disabilities experienced. This enormous variability is also found in patient presentation (**Table 1**). Some patients may be asymptomatic. Patients who have no symptoms when diagnosed have generally been identified from genetic analysis conducted because a blood relative has NF2 or presymptomatic screening.

Although the NIH criteria for NF2 require the presence of bilateral vestibular schwannomas for diagnosis, patients may first develop unilateral schwannomas as a young child with no other tumors, or adult patients may present with multiple meningiomas (cranial and spinal) and no vestibular schwannomas.[8,22] Although the NIH criteria for NF2 imply that all patients with NF2 develop bilateral vestibular schwannomas, some researchers are not convinced of this.[23] Evans and colleagues[23] based their conclusion on the observation of a possible variant form of NF2 manifesting with skin and spinal tumors in the absence of vestibular schwannomas. Nonetheless, the phenotype generally is reflective of the underlying disorder.

The natural history study of vestibular schwannomas in NF2 conducted at the House Ear Institute showed that 10 of 80 (12.5%) enrolled subjects had no symptoms at diagnosis, and 23 (28.8%) had cranial meningiomas and spinal meningiomas in addition to bilateral vestibular schwannomas. Nearly half (47.5%) had 1 vestibular schwannoma removed before enrollment. In general, the tumor resected before enrollment was removed 1.5 years after discovery, and was an average of 2.1 cm at removal. Few patients in the natural history study had spinal tumors or meningiomas removed before enrollment. The preliminary data indicate that, for this sample of subjects with NF2, the most salient medical issue is the growth of the vestibular schwannomas.

Intracranial Schwannomas

Vestibular schwannomas are the most common intracranial schwannomas associated with NF2. The most frequently identified nonvestibular schwannomas are schwannomas of CN III and V. Bilateral CN III or V schwannomas are the most common additional schwannomas seen. It is important to identify these lesions on MRI. Lower CN schwannomas may also be identified, but are much less frequently seen. A vestibular schwannoma rarely turns malignant, and sometimes unilateral vestibular

Table 1
First symptoms of neurofibromatosis 2

Symptoms	Patients (%)
Neurologic	17.5
Skin tumor	11.7
Vision loss	10.7
Asymptomatic	10.7
Tinnitus	7.8
Weakness	2.9
Vertigo	1
Other/unspecified	4.9

Adapted from Slattery WH. Neurofibromatosis 2 in otologic surgery. In: Brackmann DE, Shelton C, Arriaga MA, editors. Philadelphia: Elsevier; 2010. p. 691–701; with permission.

schwannomas regress in size altogether. Growth of the tumors does not seem to be related either to loss of heterozygosity (genetic level of analysis) or to auditory functioning (phenotype level of analysis). For this reason, it is recommended that a patient have at least yearly MRI scans to track changes in size.[24–29] All newly diagnosed patients should have a full head and spine study to stage their disease. After the disease is staged, a 6-month study is performed to determine whether the tumor is fast growing or slow growing.[30]

CN V, or trigeminal nerve, schwannomas are the most common type seen after vestibular schwannomas. Oculomotor schwannomas are the third most common schwannomas seen intracranially. Occasionally, it is difficult to distinguish whether these schwannomas have arisen from the oculomotor, trochlear, or abducent nerve, especially when the tumor arises within the cavernous sinus. Trochlear and abducent schwannomas are extremely rare, with only a handful of cases reported in the literature.

Facial nerve schwannomas may also be seen, although these are difficult to distinguish radiographically from vestibular schwannomas. Some patients present with small facial schwannomas that are encountered with large tumors in which the distinction between the facial nerve and cochlear vestibular nerve cannot be found. CN III and V schwannomas are usually slow growing and require treatment only when significant growth has occurred, or other intracranial complications are imminent.

Lower CN schwannomas can be significant in NF2 because these can lead to speech and swallowing disorders. When bilateral lower CN schwannomas or jugular foramen meningiomas are associated with these tumors, the patient may develop aspiration problems, which can cause significant morbidity. Glossopharyngeal, vagal, and hypoglossal neuropathies resulting from schwannomas on CN IX, X, and XII may lead to speech and swallowing disorders. Glossopharyngeal schwannomas are the most common schwannomas of the jugular foramen and may manifest with swallowing difficulty, which may lead to the requirement of gastrostomy feeding tubes for nutritional status.

Vagal nerve defects may contribute to swallowing difficulties related to esophageal dysmotility. Vagal nerve deficits may manifest with voice hoarseness owing to vocal cord paralysis, but the most imminent issue is aspiration, which occurs because of loss of sensory innervation to the larynx and loss of the reflexive airway protective mechanisms. Aspiration is often silent in such cases and leads to life-threatening pulmonary complications, including pneumonia. Tracheotomy may be required, leading to other potential life-threatening complications, including pulmonary infection. It is thought that lower CN neuropathies may contribute to mortality associated with NF2.

Hearing Changes in Patients with Vestibular Schwannomas

Hearing loss is well documented as the most common presenting symptom in patients who have vestibular schwannomas.[31–40] Auditory changes over time in patients with vestibular schwannoma are less well known. Rosenberg[41] studied the natural history of 80 patients with non-NF2 unilateral vestibular schwannomas for an average of 4.4 years and found a positive correlation between tumor growth and worsening pure tone average. However, there was no statistically significant correlation between positive tumor growth and speech discrimination, change in ABR, and bithermal caloric electronystagmography testing result over time.

Lalwani and colleagues[42] reported that pure tone pattern speech receptive thresholds and word recognition scores were significantly worse in patients with NF2 who had a mild form of NF2 and large tumors compared with patients with mild NF2 with small tumors. Loss of acoustic reflexes and prolonged wave III and V were also associated with larger tumors. In contrast, patients with severe NF2 showed no relationship among tumor size and pure tone levels, speech discrimination thresholds, or word recognition scores. The lack of association may have been caused by complete loss of hearing in patients with severe NF2 at the time of the assessment. The larger tumors were also associated with prolonged ABR waves III and V latencies. No data across time were reported. In general, hearing is progressively impaired with increasing growth of vestibular schwannomas necessitating surgical intervention or medical treatments in patients with NF2.

The natural history study evaluated hearing changes prospectively in 63 patients newly diagnosed with NF, and found that hearing was stable after diagnosis. During the first 2 years after diagnosis, 27% of patients had a significant change in their hearing, and 73% had very stable hearing during the 2-year period. Patients with a family history of NF2 had more stable hearing after an initial diagnosis compared with patients without a family history. Patients with a family history are usually diagnosed at a younger age; the stability of hearing in this group may represent the younger age group. The better the hearing in the newly diagnosed patients, the more stable the hearing. Hearing changes did not vary between ears, with each ear acting independently.[43]

OTHER TUMOR TYPES IN NEUROFIBROMATOSIS TYPE 2
Meningiomas

NF2 has been associated with multiple central nervous system tumors, the most common of which are intracranial meningiomas (**Fig. 2**).[2] Nearly all patients with NF2 develop these tumors in time. Fifty percent of patients with NF2 present with schwannomas and meningiomas; 90% present with spine tumors in addition to schwannomas. The presence of more than 1 type of tumor in a patient usually indicates a more aggressive disease course. The co-occurrence of vestibular schwannomas and meningiomas has been linked to a synergistic effect of increase in growth rate of the schwannoma and the meningioma beyond that expected of a sporadic schwannoma or meningioma.[44,45] Despite the high number of patients with multiple tumors initially, most meningiomas and spinal tumors are asymptomatic and are first seen on MRI. In addition, multiple skin tumors may be found in patients with NF2 (**Table 2**).

Meningiomas are monitored in NF2 unless they are large. Growing meningiomas may be surgically removed. Growing meningiomas may result in increased intracranial pressure, intractable headaches, hydrocephalus, and seizure disorders.

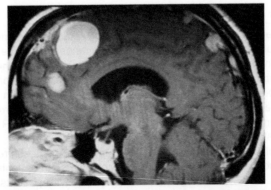

Fig. 2. Multiple meningiomas can be seen in severe forms of NF2. Meningiomas may occur throughout the cranium and skull base area.

Table 2 Tumor type	
Tumor Type	**Patients (%)**
Bilateral VS	99
Skin	50
Meningioma	46
Spinal	60

Abbreviation: VS, vestibular schwannoma.
Adapted from Slattery WH. Neurofibromatosis 2 in otologic surgery. In: Brackmann DE, Shelton C, Arriaga MA, editors. Philadelphia: Elsevier; 2010. p. 691–701; with permission.

Spinal Tumors

Various spinal tumors may occur in patients with NF2, and can be found in the cervical, thoracic, and lumbar region. These tumors are categorized further as either extramedullary or intramedullary tumors depending on their presentation relative to the spinal cord. Extramedullary tumors are commonly schwannomas or meningiomas, whereas intramedullary tumors are often ependymomas, but these can be astrocytomas or schwannomas.[2] Spinal tumors are often numerous small tumors in the cauda equina. Tumors located in the cervical or thoracic region are usually solitary tumors, and these may grow to cause spinal cord compression. These tumors may have a solid or cystic component similar to schwannomas and meningiomas seen intracranially. These tumors may extend out of the spinal foramen into the soft tissue, causing spinal cord compression.[2]

As each NF2-related tumor grows and exerts pressure on surrounding structures, treatment encompasses surgical resection, radiation therapy, or both. Another treatment choice early in the disease course is surgical decompression, in which space is created for the growing tumor, relieving the pressure of the tumor against the nerve. Continued growth of spinal tumors causes loss of motion, numbness, tingling, and eventually paralysis. Some patients (2% to 3% of patients)[2] present with numbness or tingling in their arms or legs. Almost 30% of patients with NF2 have surgery to remove spinal tumors, but the progression of spinal tumors associated with NF2 is not well described. At this time, the presence of vestibular schwannoma in NF2 and the consequences of not treating them are well known, and these tumors may be the most debilitating.

Eye Findings

Patients with NF2 also tend to develop cortical and posterior subcapsular cataracts, which can lead to blindness (see **Table 1**).[2] Retinal hamartomas have been observed in a few cases,[2,4] but are not as frequent.

Skin Tumors

Skin tumors can be found in many patients with NF2. These tumors are usually small schwannomas of peripheral nerve origin. They are usually asymptomatic and are commonly missed on physical examination unless the patient brings it to the attention of the clinician. These tumors are only removed if they present a cosmetic problem or cause a functional impairment, such when found on the hand or foot.

Treatment Options for Vestibular Schwannomas in Neurofibromatosis Type 2

The treatment options for patients with bilateral vestibular schwannomas vary considerably because of the wide variety of tumor sizes and clinical presentations.

Associated symptoms (brainstem compression or hydrocephalus), loss of useful hearing, and the status of other intracranial tumors all must be considered when discussing treatment intervention.

Hearing Preservation

Patients who present with bilateral small tumors (<2 cm in greatest diameter) and good hearing may be candidates for hearing preservation procedures. In these patients, total tumor removal is attempted on the side of the larger tumor or on the side with worse hearing. If hearing is successfully preserved on the first side, contralateral tumor removal may be attempted 6 months later. Hearing preservation rates for small unilateral tumors have approached 70%.[40] However, the results in patients with NF2 seem to be worse than the results reported in patients with unilateral vestibular schwannomas.[46] Doyle and Shelton[47] found that 67% of patients with NF2 underwent hearing preservation surgery using the middle fossa approach, and 38% of those had serviceable hearing postoperatively. Improvements in the middle fossa surgical approach were introduced in 1992 that led to a significant improvement in the outcomes of NF2 tumor removal. A more recent review of 18 patients with NF2 who had middle fossa removal of their tumors reported that approximately 50% of patients had hearing preserved at the preoperative level; this compares with 25% in the previous study. The overall ability to preserve any hearing was still close to 68%.[48] The results of this series have led to a more aggressive attempt to preserve hearing in patients with NF2. Patients who present with small tumors and good hearing are now routinely offered an attempt at hearing preservation. Long-term follow-up is still needed in patients with NF2 because additional tumors may arise in the facial or cochlear nerves.

We have published our results treating children with NF2 with small tumors and good hearing. This retrospective chart review reported on 35 children with NF2 who had undergone middle fossa resection (47 surgeries) between 1992 and 2004. In 55% of surgeries, hearing of less than or equal to 70 dB pure tone average was maintained postoperatively. It is now our practice to perform middle fossa resection in children with NF2, and the sooner in the disease process the better. Our results indicate that hearing and facial nerve function can be successfully preserved using this approach. Factors to consider include patient age; severity of additional NF2-related symptoms; and obtaining high-quality, thin-slice MR images before surgery. Bilateral middle fossa resection after hearing preservation on the first side is also successful and potentially preserves hearing in both ears.[49]

Observation Without Surgical Intervention

Observation without surgical intervention is the most common treatment option used in patients with NF2 and is used when a small tumor is present in a patient with only 1 hearing ear or when bilateral tumors are too large for hearing preservation procedures. The patient is assessed routinely to ensure that brainstem compression or hydrocephalus does not result. Initially, MRI is performed 6 months after diagnosis, and then annual MRI scans are performed to document tumor size and determine whether intervention is required. Surgical intervention is considered if life-threatening complications occur, the tumors become excessively large (increasing the perioperative morbidity), or the hearing becomes unserviceable.

Middle fossa craniotomy and IAC decompression without tumor removal allow the tumor to grow without causing compression of CN VII and VIII. This procedure is recommended when progression of hearing loss occurs in a patient who is being observed. The bone surrounding the IAC is removed extensively, allowing the entire tumor and CN VII and VIII complex to be decompressed. The tumor is not removed because this may increase the risk of hearing loss. Stabilization and improvement of hearing may occur after this procedure. In our review of 49 patients who underwent middle fossa craniotomy with decompression of the internal auditory canal at the House Clinic, preoperative American Academy of Otolaryngology – Head and Neck Surgery hearing class was preserved in 90% of patients in the immediate postoperative period and approximately two-thirds of patients at 1 year from surgery.[50] The average duration of hearing preservation was slightly more than 2 years, with some patients showing hearing preservation for periods up to 10 years.

Retrosigmoid Craniotomy with Partial Removal

Retrosigmoid craniotomy with partial removal in patients with NF2 carries a significant risk because the cochlear fibers are dispersed throughout the tumor, in contrast with unilateral vestibular schwannomas (**Fig. 3**). The risk of hearing loss with partial removal is much higher, and this procedure is typically not recommended.

Non–hearing Preservation

The most common surgical procedure performed in patients with NF2 is the non–hearing preservation, translabyrinthine/suboccipital approach and total tumor removal.

Translabyrinthine/Suboccipital Approach and Total Tumor Removal

Most patients present when either the tumor is too large for hearing preservation or the hearing loss is already at a significant level and hearing preservation is not considered. This approach is used for patients with large tumors who have brainstem compression even if serviceable hearing exists. The translabyrinthine or suboccipital craniotomy approaches may be used for this procedure. However, the risk of a recurrent tumor is slightly higher with the suboccipital approach and with inexperienced surgeons because residual tumor is often left in the lateral aspect of the IAC.

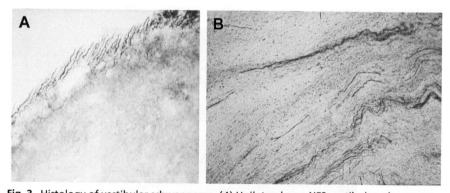

Fig. 3. Histology of vestibular schwannoma. (*A*) Unilateral non-NF2 vestibular schwannoma. Typical schwannoma stain with Bodian silver stain, which stains only the nerve fiber so the schwannoma cells are not evident. However, the fibers on the surface of the tumor are visible. (*B*) Another Bodian silver stain with black strands embedded within the tumor, representing the nerve fibers invaded by the tumor. This invasion is different from that seen in non-NF2 solitary vestibular schwannomas. Non-NF2 solitary tumors invade the aggregates of cells and push the fibers aside, rather than invading between the fibers. NF2 vestibular schwannomas are histologically different from non-NF2 sporadic, unilateral tumors. (*Courtesy of* Fred H. Linthicum Jr, MD, House Research Institute Temporal Bone Histopathology Laboratory, Los Angeles, CA; with permission.)

Auditory Brainstem Implant

The auditory brainstem implant (ABI) was developed at the House Ear Institute to allow electric stimulation of the cochlear nucleus after bilateral vestibular schwannoma removal. The device is placed on the brainstem (**Fig. 4**) during translabyrinthine vestibular schwannoma removal. This device is indicated in individuals who have no serviceable hearing and are undergoing vestibular schwannoma removal. Most patients obtain enhanced communication skills with the device. The ABI can be placed with the first tumor removal even when useful hearing is still present on the contralateral ear. This procedure is recommended when the patient has bilateral large tumors and the chance of losing hearing in the nonsurgery ear is great. Another advantage of first-side surgery is that the patient has the opportunity to have 2 ABIs, resulting in an overall better outcome.

Cochlear Implants in Neurofibromatosis Type 2

The variability of ABI results between patients has led us to reexamine the utility of cochlear implantation for auditory rehabilitation in patients with NF2. In the presence of an intact cochlear nerve, cochlear implantation offers a viable and, in our experience in properly selected patients, often successful approach for hearing rehabilitation. The use of electrical promontory stimulation to determine the presence of intact and functional cochlear nerve fibers aids in determining cochlear implant candidacy and selection of the appropriate ear. At least 10 patients have been reported as receiving cochlear implants after they lost hearing following stereotactic radiotherapy.[51] All patients had tumor growth controlled with radiotherapy. Hearing outcomes in this select group of patients with their cochlear implants were considered successful in most patients. Our unpublished experience at the House Clinic shows that this approach can be successful and is in agreement with the current published literature.

Stereotactic Irradiation

Stereotactic irradiation has been recommended for some patients with NF2, but its use must be carefully considered because radiation exposure may induce or accelerate tumors in patients with inactivated tumor suppressor genes. It has been reported

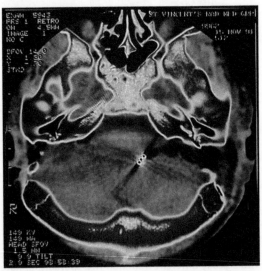

Fig. 4. CT scan showing placement of an ABI within the lateral recess of the fourth ventricle on the right.

that at least 5 of 106 patients with NF2 who underwent radiotherapy developed radiation-induced malignancies and that, although patients with NF2 represent approximately 7% of irradiated patients, nearly 50% of reports of malignant degeneration occur in the context of NF2.[52,53]

Many algorithms have been proposed as treatment plans, but none are widely accepted among NF2 specialists. The range of treatment options is large; larger than for any other nervous system tumor. The potential benefits of treatment are great (hearing preservation), but the potential risks are also significant, and the riskiest procedures have the greatest potential benefit. Note that the risk of hearing loss is substantial with radiotherapy. Mathieu and colleagues[54] noted 1-year, 2-year, and 5-year actuarial serviceable hearing preservation rates of 73%, 59%, and 48% respectively in patients with NF2 who underwent stereotactic radiosurgery for vestibular schwannoma. Often patients have a window of opportunity when they can choose a risky but potentially beneficial procedure; once the window closes, they cannot go back. Patients, families, and care providers need to know the natural history of these tumors to make rational recommendations and decisions regarding these treatment options. In addition, noninvasive and tumor-related markers of behavior need to be identified that can tailor further anticipatory guidance for each patient.

Drug Therapy

Current investigations into drug therapies for NF2 seek to target multiple intracellular signaling pathways that interact with the NF2 protein, including the phosphatidylinositol 3 kinase/Akt, Raf/MEK/ERK, and mTOR pathways as well as integrin/focal adhesion kinase/Src/Ras signaling cascades, platelet-derived growth factor receptor beta, and vascular endothelial growth factor (VEGF) pathways.[4] Current investigations of drugs such as erlotinib, lapatinib, and bevacizumab continue to evaluate their efficacy in treatment of NF-related tumors. Much attention has been focused recently on anti-VEGF therapies, including bevacizumab and Avastin. Although preclinical studies have shown much interest, current clinical investigations of Avastin in patients with NF2 remain ongoing.[55,56] Clinical trials are currently open and investigating bevacizumab, lapatinib, and rapamycin to stop growth of NF2 vestibular schwannomas. Early results of drug therapies have been promising, but long-term studies are needed to show benefit. As an example, erlotinib was reported to be effective in a case report, but a larger study showed that it was not effective and many patients experienced side effects.[57,58] Some patients with NF2 have participated in experimental new drug therapy only to develop severe side effects. Drug therapy as a therapeutic option may become standard therapy, but well-controlled long-term studies are needed before it can be routinely recommended.

MANAGEMENT OF NEUROFIBROMATOSIS TYPE 2

Initial evaluation of a patient with NF1 can be complex because this is a multisystem disease. An inadequate diagnosis may render a patient impaired because early diagnosis and treatment may have prevented further impairments. Patients with NF2 may typically see many different physicians, each with experience in a different field of expertise. Patients with NF2 require 1 physician to lead the treatment team (a case manager, as it were) to ensure comprehensive care. A neuro-otologist, geneticist, neurosurgeon, or neurologist may function as the lead physician, depending on the NF2 center.

A comprehensive battery of tests is necessary for tumor detection and adequate staging. The initial MRI study showing the presence of bilateral vestibular schwannomas may be inadequate for tumor follow-up. A cranial MRI scan may not have included the IACs, or a spine series may have focused on only 1 segment of the spine. MRI with gadolinium and thin cuts through the IAC is necessary for the head. Particular attention is focused on the IACs, cavernous sinus, and jugular foramen areas. Any CN may have tumor formation and should have complete imaging. Auditory assessment is necessary to determine the extent of hearing impairment. At a minimum, this assessment consists of a standard audiogram, with air and bone pure tone thresholds, and speech testing. Some centers prefer additional testing with ABR to assess cochlear nerve function. ABR testing is particularly helpful when considering a hearing preservation procedure. Electronystagmography testing has benefit in determining tumor location; however, its utility for clinical assessment is still under investigation.

A complete neurologic examination is required for individuals with suspected NF2. The standard neurologic assessment of dermatomes and muscle strength is required for assessment of potential spinal cord impairment. CN testing may find subtle abnormalities for which the patient has slowly compensated. In addition, patients may not even be aware of their own impairment, particularly of the lower CNs.

A complete MRI spinal cord survey is required to identify tumors within the spine. The use of spine screening is still under investigation for all patients with NF2. Patients with a significant tumor burden, a family history of spine tumors, or spinal tumor symptoms should have a spine series. A spine series is required in all symptomatic patients.

A neuro-ophthalmologic examination is required for all patients with NF2. The potential for deafness in these individuals requires that everything be done to preserve vision. A slit-lamp examination is required. It is preferable that a patient be evaluated by an ophthalmologist familiar with NF2.

The initial comprehensive evaluation consists, at a minimum, of MRI of the IAC with gadolinium, auditory assessment, and physical examination. A comprehensive examination includes the previously mentioned MRI with the addition of a full spine series, an ABR test, and an ophthalmologic examination.

The timing of follow-up studies is currently inconsistent among NF2 specialty centers. We recommend repeat testing at 6 months and then yearly testing consisting of MRI of the head and spine, neurology examination, and audiometric testing. When the growth rate from the tumors has been determined, some of these tests may be spread out over time. Spinal tumors tend to be slow growing, and after diagnosis may be imaged every 1 to 5 years. The potential for new tumor formation exists, especially in patients with severe disease, and it is important that this information be conveyed to patients with NF1 so that comprehensive follow-up may occur.

Genetic Testing

Identification of the NF2 gene on chromosome 22 has made genetic testing possible. It is recommended that patients with NF2 see a genetic counselor to discuss the hereditary consequences of this disease. All patients with NF2 should be given the opportunity to have genetic testing performed. The preferred method is testing of fresh tumor tissue, which is usually accomplished when the first tumor is removed and the tumor can be frozen and sent to a clinical laboratory that is certified to perform the genetic test. Genetic blood screening is able to identify the defect on the NF2 gene in approximately 70% to 75% of patients with a known diagnosis of NF2. If the defect is identified, potential family members may be screened. However, mutation screening may not reveal the causative mutation. Tumor analysis can play a role in genetic testing for the offspring of sporadic patients. Analysis of the tumor can be used to take a targeted approach to analysis of the blood sample. Once the genetic mutation is identified, screening of at-risk relatives can be performed with only a blood test. If the gene is not identified, blood screening of family members cannot be performed. The use of blood screening for patients without a diagnosis or with a suspected diagnosis of NF2 is not recommended. New mutations in patients with mild presentation are most likely missense mutations, which are difficult to identify by genetic testing. If both mutational events are identified in the NF2 gene in the tumor and neither is present in the blood, then the patient is likely a mosaic for one of these mutations.[4] Because 25% to 30% of patients with NF2 are thought to be mosaic, frozen tumors should be taken at the time of operation (with patient consent) for genetic testing.

SUMMARY

Care of patients with NF2 requires knowledge of all tumors and symptoms involved with the disorder. It is recommended that patients receive care in a center with expertise in NF2. The role of the neuro-otologist in this care is determined by the specialty center.

REFERENCES

1. Guttmann DH, Aylswort A, Carey JC, et al. The diagnostic evaluation and multi-disciplinary management of NF1 and NF2. JAMA 1997;278:51–7.
2. Asthagiri AR, Parry DM, Butman JA, et al. Neurofibromatosis type 2. Lancet 2009; 373(9679):1974–86.
3. Evans DG, Howard E, Giblin C, et al. Birth incidence and prevalence of tumor-prone syndromes: estimates from a UK family genetic register service. Am J Med Genet A 2010;152A:327–32.
4. Evans DG. Neurofibromatosis type 2 (NF2): a clinical and molecular review. Orphanet J Rare Dis 2009;4:16.
5. Ruggieri M, Huson SM. The clinical and diagnostic implications of mosaicism in the neurofibromatoses. Neurology 2001;56:1433–43.
6. Baser ME, Mautner VF, Ragge NK, et al. Presymptomatic diagnosis of neurofibromatosis 2 using linked genetic markers, neuroimaging, and ocular examinations. Neurology 1996;47:1269–77.
7. Bijlsma EK, Merel P, Fleury P, et al. Family with neurofibromatosis type 2 and autosomal dominant hearing loss: identification of carriers of the mutated NF2 gene. Hum Genet 1995;96:1–5.
8. Mautner VF, Baser ME, Kluwe L. Phenotype variability in two families with novel splice-site and frameshift NF2 mutations. Hum Genet 1996;98:203–6.
9. Sainio M, Strachan T, Blomstedt G, et al. Presymptomatic DNA and MRI diagnosis of neurofibromatosis 2 with mild clinical course in an extended pedigree. Neurology 1995;45:1314–22.
10. Welling DB. Clinical manifestations of mutations in the neurofibromatosis type 2 gene in vestibular schwannomas (acoustic neuromas). Laryngoscope 1998; 108:178–89.
11. Shelton C, Brackmann DE, House WF. Middle fossa approach. In: Brackmann DE, Shelton C, Arriaga MA, editors. Otologic surgery. 3rd edition. Philadelphia: Elsevier; 2010. p. 581–9.
12. Antinheimo J, Sankila R, Carpen O, et al. Population-based analysis of sporadic and type 2 neurofibromatosis-associated meningiomas and schwannomas. Neurology 2000;54:71–6.
13. Rouleau GA, Wertelecki W, Haines JL, et al. Genetic linkage of bilateral acoustic neurofibromatosis to a DNA marker on chromosome 22. Nature 1987;329:246–8.

14. Rouleau GA, Merel P, Lutchman M, et al. Alteration in a new gene encoding a putative membrane-organizing protein causes neurofibromatosis type 2. Nature 1993;363:515–21.

15. Trofatter JA, MacCollin MM, Rutter JL, et al. A novel moesin-, ezrin-, radixin-like gene is a candidate for the neurofibromatosis type 2 tumor suppressor. Cell 1993;72:791–800.

16. Merel P, Haong-Xuan K, Sanson M, et al. Predominant occurrence of somatic mutations of the NF2 gene in meningiomas and schwannomas. Genes Chromosomes Cancer 1995;13:211–6.

17. Merel P, Hoang-Xuan K, Sanson M, et al. Screening for germ-line mutations in the NF2 gene. Genes Chromosomes Cancer 1995;12:117–27.

18. Welling DB, Guida M, Goll F, et al. Mutational spectrum in the neurofibromatosis type 2 gene in sporadic and familial schwannomas. Hum Genet 1996;98:189–93.

19. Wu CL, Thakker N, Neary W, et al. Differential diagnosis of type 2 neurofibromatosis: molecular discrimination of NF2 and sporadic vestibular schwannomas. J Med Genet 1998;35:973–7.

20. Irving RM, Harada T, Moffat DA, et al. Somatic neurofibromatosis type 2 gene mutations and growth characteristics in vestibular schwannoma. Am J Otol 1997;18:754–60.

21. Cushing H. Bilateral acoustic tumors, generalized neurofibromatosis and the meningeal endotheliomata. Tumors of the nervous acoustics and the syndrome of the cerebellopontine angle. Philadelphia: Saunders; 1963. 1917 original edition.

22. Mautner VF, Lindenau M, Koppen J, et al. Type 2 neurofibromatosis without acoustic neuroma. Zentralbl Neurochir 1995;56:83–7.

23. Evans DG, Lye R, Neary W, et al. Probability of bilateral disease in people presenting with a unilateral vestibular schwannoma. J Neurol Neurosurg Psychiatry 1999;66:764–7.

24. Mathies C, Samii M, Krebs S. Management of vestibular schwannomas (acoustic neuromas): radiological features in 202 cases—their value for diagnosis and their predictive importance. Neurosurgery 1997;40:469–81.

25. Burkey JM, Rizer FM, Schuring AG, et al. Acoustic reflexes, auditory brainstem response, and MRI in the evaluation of acoustic neuromas. Laryngoscope 1996;106:839–41.

26. Levine SC, Antonelli PJ, Le CT, et al. Relative value of diagnostic tests for small acoustic neuromas. Am J Otol 1991;12:341–6.

27. Lhullier FM, Doyon DL, Halimi PM, et al. Magnetic resonance imaging of acoustic neuromas: pitfalls and differential diagnosis. Neuroradiology 1992;34:144–9.

28. Long SA, Arriaga M, Nelson RA. Acoustic neuroma volume: MRI-based calculations and clinical implications. Laryngoscope 1993;103:1093–6.

29. Modugno GC, Pirodda A, Ferri GG, et al. Small acoustic neuromas: monitoring the growth rate by MRI. Acta Neurochir 1999;141:1063–7.

30. Irving RM, Moffat DA, Hardy DG, et al. A molecular, clinical, and immunohistochemical study of vestibular schwannoma. Otolaryngol Head Neck Surg 1997;116:426–30.

31. Strasnick B, Glasscock ME III, Haynes D, et al. The natural history of untreated acoustic neuromas. Laryngoscope 1994;104:1115–9.

32. Fucci MJ, Buchman CA, Brackmann DE, et al. Acoustic tumor growth: implications for treatment choices. Am J Otol 1999;20:495–9.

33. Brackmann DE, Owens RM, Friedman RA, et al. Prognostic factors for hearing preservation in vestibular schwannoma surgery. Am J Otol 1999;20:495–9.

34. Briggs RJ, Brackmann DE, Baser ME, et al. Comprehensive management of bilateral acoustic neuromas: current perspectives. Arch Otolaryngol Head Neck Surg 1994;120:1307–14.

35. Doyle KJ, Nelson RA. Bilateral acoustic neuromas (NF2). In: House WF, Luetje CM, Doyle KJ, editors. Acoustic tumors: diagnosis and management. San Diego (CA): Singular Publishing Group; 1997.

36. Evans DG, Huson SM, Donnai D, et al. A genetic study of type 2 neurofibromatosis in the United Kingdom. I: Prevalence, mutation rate, fitness, and confirmation of maternal transmission effect on severity. J Med Genet 1992;29:841–6.

37. Gadre AK, Kwartler JA, Brackmann DE, et al. Middle fossa decompression of the internal auditory canal in acoustic neuroma surgery: a therapeutic alternative. Laryngoscope 1990;100:948–52.

38. Kesterson L, Shelton C, Dressler L, et al. Clinical behavior of acoustic tumors: a flow cytometric analysis. Arch Otolaryngol Head Neck Surg 1993;119:269–71.

39. Saunders JE, Luxford WM, Devgan KK, et al. Sudden hearing loss in acoustic neuroma patients. Otolaryngol Head Neck Surg 1995;113:23–31.

40. Slattery WH III, Brackmann DE, Hitselberger W. Middle fossa approach for hearing preservation with acoustic neuromas. Am J Otol 1997;18:596–601.

41. Rosenberg SI. Natural history of acoustic neuromas. Laryngoscope 2000;110: 497–508.

42. Lalwani AK, Abaza MM, Makariou EV, et al. Audiologic presentation of vestibular schwannoma in neurofibromatosis type 2. Am J Otol 1998;19:352–7.

43. Masuda A, Fischer LM, Oppenheimer ML, et al. Hearing changes after diagnosis in neurofibromatosis type 2. Otol Neurotol 2004;25(2):150–4.

44. Pallini R, Tancredi A, Cassalbore P, et al. Neurofibromatosis type 2: growth stimulation of mixed acoustic schwannoma by concurrent adjacent meningioma: possible role of growth factors. Case report. J Neurosurg 1998;89:149–54.

45. Antinheimo J, Haappasalo H, Haltia M, et al. Proliferation potential and histological features in neurofibromatosis 2-associated and sporadic meningiomas. J Neurosurg 1997;87:610–4.

46. Slattery WH III, Brackmann DE. Hearing preservation and restoration in CPA tumor surgery. Neurosurgery 1997;Q7:169–82.

47. Doyle KJ, Shelton C. Hearing preservation in bilateral acoustic neuroma surgery. Am J Otol 1993;14:562–5.

48. Slattery WH, Brackmann DE, Hitzelburger W. Hearing preservation in NF-2. Am J Otol 1998;19:638–43.

49. Slattery WH, Fischer LM, Hitzelburger W, et al. Hearing preservation surgery for NF-2 related vestibular schwannomas in pediatric patients. J Neurosurg 2007; 106:255–60.

50. Slattery WH, Hoa M, Bonne N, et al. Middle fossa decompression for hearing preservation: a review of institutional results and indications. Otol Neurotol 2011;32(6):1017–24.

51. Trotter MI, Briggs RJ. Cochlear implantation in neurofibromatosis type 2 after radiation therapy. Otol Neurotol 2010;31:216–9.

52. Baser ME, Evans DG, Jackler RK, et al. Neurofibromatosis 2, radiosurgery and malignant nervous system tumours. Br J Cancer 2000;82(4):998.

53. Evans DG, Birch JM, Ramsden RT, et al. Malignant transformation and new primary tumours after therapeutic radiation for benign disease: substantial risks in certain tumour prone syndromes. J Med Genet 2006;43:289–94.

54. Mathieu D, Kondziolka D, Flickinger JC, et al. Stereotactic radiosurgery for vestibular schwannomas in patients with neurofibromatosis type 2: an analysis of tumor

control, complications, and hearing preservation rates. Neurosurgery 2007;60: 460–70.

55. Wong HK, Lahdenranta J, Kamoun WS, et al. Anti-vascular endothelial growth factor therapies as a novel therapeutic approach to treating neurofibromatosis-related tumors. Cancer Res 2010;70(9):3483–93.

56. Plotkin SR, Stemmer-Rachamimov AO, Barker FG 2nd, et al. Hearing improvement after bevacizumab in patients with neurofibromatosis type 2. N Engl J Med 2009;361(4):358–67.

57. Plotkin SR, Singh MA, O'Donnell CC, et al. Audiologic and radiographic response of NF2-related vestibular schwannoma to erlotinib therapy. Nat Clin Pract Oncol 2008;5(8):487–91.

58. Plotkin SR, Halpin C, McKenna MJ, et al. Erlotinib for progressive vestibular schwannoma in neurofibromatosis 2 patients. Otol Neurotol 2010;31(7):1135–43.

Nonschwannoma Tumors of the Cerebellopontine Angle

David R. Friedmann, MD[a], Bartosz Grobelny, MD[b],
John G. Golfinos, MD[b], J. Thomas Roland Jr, MD[c],*

KEYWORDS

- Cerebellopontine angle tumors • Posterior fossa meningioma • Epidermoid
- Lipoma • Endolymphatic sac tumors • Hemangioblastoma

KEY POINTS

- Vestibular schwannoma (VS), meningioma, epidermoid, and lipoma account for 95% of cerebellopontine angle (CPA) lesions.
- There is wide differential of rarer lesions of the CPA, including benign and malignant lesions.
- Many of these lesions may mimic schwannomas except for subtle imaging findings underlying the importance of their careful review.
- Management of CPA pathology may include single- or multimodality treatment, including observation, microsurgical resection, and stereotactic radiation therapy.

Videos of a presigmoid retrolabrynthine approach to a cerebellopontine meningioma and a transpetrosal approach to an intracranial epidermoid accompany this article at http://www.oto.theclinics.com/

INTRODUCTION

Fewer than 10% of intracranial neoplasms involve the CPA in adults although this number is less than 1% in children.[1] Although VSs are the most common lesion of the CPA (70%–90%), other pathology may present in this location. Meningiomas are the second most common lesion, occurring between 5% and 15% of cases,

Disclosures: None.
[a] Division of Otology/Neurotology and Skull Base Surgery, Department of Otolaryngology-Head & Neck Surgery, New York University School of Medicine, 550 1st Ave, Skirball Suite 7q, New York, NY 10016, USA; [b] Department of Neurosurgery, New York University School of Medicine, 550 1st Ave, Skirball Suite 8s, New York, NY 10016, USA; [c] Department of Otolaryngology-Head & Neck Surgery, New York University School of Medicine, 550 1st Ave, Skirball Suite 7q, New York, NY 10016, USA
* Corresponding author.
E-mail address: tom.roland@nyumc.org

Otolaryngol Clin N Am 48 (2015) 461–475
http://dx.doi.org/10.1016/j.otc.2015.02.006
0030-6665/15/$ – see front matter © 2015 Elsevier Inc. All rights reserved.

Abbreviations	
CPA	Cerebellopontine angle
CSF	Cerebrospinal fluid
ELST	Endolymphatic sac tumor
VHL	von Hippel-Landau
VS	Vestibular schwannoma

followed by epidermoids and lipomas. A wide differential of rarer lesions compose the remainder, some of which develop directly in the CPA, whereas others may extend from neighboring structures. Diagnosis may be made from the clinical history as well as radiologic features (**Table 1**).

NONSCHWANNOMATOUS LESIONS OF CEREBELLOPONTINE ANGLE
Meningioma

Meningiomas, which develop from arachnoid cap cells in the dura, are the second most common tumor in the CPA, comprising approximately 10% of lesions in this location. Of all locations, approximately 10% of meningiomas are found in the CPA.[2] These can have origins in the dura around the internal auditory canal, Meckel cave, jugular foramen, jugular tubercle, suprameatal tubercle, sigmoid sinus, torcula, the superior or inferior petrosal sinuses, porus acusticus, and clivus although most commonly they originate from the posterior petrous dura.[3] They tend to be benign tumors that displace local structures at the tumor's periphery as opposed to infiltrating, although they may be adherent. There is a female predominance in CPA meningiomas, as there is with those in other locations.

As opposed to the presentation of VSs, audiovestibular symptoms (hearing loss, tinnitus, and dysequilibrium) are less frequent and of shorter duration with cerebellopontine meningiomas.[4] Nevertheless, audiovestibular symptoms predominate. Facial pain, which is rarely seen in VS patients, can present in up to 30% of cerebellopontine meningiomas. Dysesthesias and facial spasms can be presenting signs as well. Cerebellar signs are frequently seen in these meningiomas compared with VSs, in which they are rare.[5]

Table 1
Differential of lesions of cerebellopontine angle with imaging characteristics

Tumor Type	Radiographic Characteristics
VSs, hemangioblastoma	T1 iso/hypointense, T2 isointense, enhance with contrast (vascular flow voids for hemangioblastoma)
Meningioma, hemangiopericytomas	Uniformly enhancing, broad petrous base, hyperostosis of underlying bone, possible calcifications
Epidermoid	CSF-like intensity on CT and MRI T1, T2 sequences demonstrate restriction on diffusion sequences
Lipomas	Hyperintense on T1, do not enhance, lose their signal on fat-suppression sequences
ELSTs	T1 hyperintense, heterogenous enhancement with contrast
Glomus tumors/paragangliomas	T1 hypointense, T2 hyperintense, enhance with gadolinium
Arachnoid cyst, granulation	CSF-like intensity on CT and all MRI sequences, may erode bone

Radiologic diagnosis of cerebellopontine meningioma is made typically with gadolinium-enhanced MRI of the brain. They are uniformly enhancing, hemispheric, semilunar masses with a broad petrous base to which they are attached they are usually asymmetric to the internal auditory canal.[6] Classically, an enhancing dural tail can be appreciated at the tumor's margin (**Fig. 1**). On CT, potential calcifications or hyperostosis of the surrounding bone can be appreciated. Sometimes it may be hard to differentiate between meningiomas and schwannomas in the CPA. One study has shown 94% sensitivity and 100% specificity differentiating meningiomas from VSs based on lack of microhemorrhages on T2-weighted gradient echo.[7]

Treatment of meningiomas depends on the symptomatology and goals of treatment. An asymptomatic meningioma can be followed with serial MRI scans to assess for growth. Serial scanning and observation may also be used in patients with advanced age or comorbidities that preclude surgery. In these cases, stereotactic radiosurgery may also be considered. If surgical resection is planned, the goal is maximum safe removal of the tumor, avoiding injury to involved cranial nerves, with wide excision of the dural attachment as well as resection of hyperostotic bone, which can contain infiltrative tumor.

As with VSs, the surgical approaches for these tumors include the retrosigmoid, translabyrinthine, and middle fossa craniotomies. The most common approach used is the retrosigmoid, which offers access to the CPA when hearing preservation is attempted. The translabyrinthine approach is another viable option, with an advantage of less cerebellar retraction during surgery but inevitably sacrifices any residual hearing. This approach may be used in patients with tumors that fill the entire internal acoustic meatus or patients in whom hearing is already poor or not salvageable.[2] The

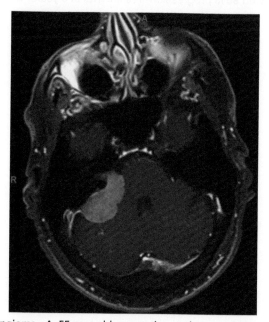

Fig. 1. CPA meningioma. A 55-year-old man who underwent MRI with contrast. This T1-enhanced image demonstrates a dural-based mass in the right CPA. There is a dural tail and invasion of the internal acoustic meatus. This was found to be an atypical (WHO grade II) meningioma.

middle fossa approach is generally not useful because it is not appropriate in tumors that extend more than 1 cm out of the internal acoustic meatus. A subtemporal/transpetrosal approach has also been used. It facilitates exposure particularly for meningiomas that extend either anterior or superior to the interior auditory meatus, along the petroclival region. Advantages with this approach include early devascularization of the tumor, small amounts of brain retraction, preservation of the vein of Labbé, and access to both supra- and infratentorial compartments.[3] Combined approaches also may be advantageous depending on tumor location.

Posterior fossa meningiomas adjacent to the endolymphatic duct may present with a specific symptom complex of vertigo, sensorineural hearing loss, tinnitus, and aural fullness (**Fig. 2**). Such patients may be misdiagnosed as having Meniere's disease. The authors have previously described management of these particular lesions.[8] Surgical resection via a retrolabyrinthine or retrosigmoid craniotomy may result in successful preservation of hearing and improvement in vestibular symptoms (Video 1).

Outcomes from surgical resection of meningiomas vary depending on tumor location and size. In recent series, gross total resections were achieved in 45% to 86%. Mortality ranged between 0% and 5%. Permanent post operative facial weakness occurred in 6% to 11% with as many as 30% having postoperative facial paresis. Swallowing problems occurred in 2% to 12%.[3] Hearing declined in 17% of patients in hearing preservation surgeries, although 1 large study found 91% of functional hearing preservation in their series.[3]

Stereotactic radiosurgery may be used for cerebellopontine meningiomas, either primary or adjuvant treatment. Good long-term control and a low side-effect profile has been demonstrated.[9] One study examined radiosurgery in CPA meningiomas, specifically. It showed 95% progression-free survival at 5 years, with 31% of patients

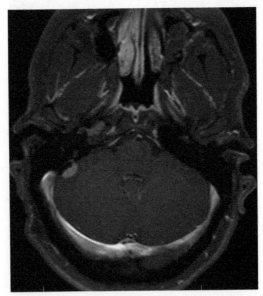

Fig. 2. Meningioma adjacent to endolymphatic sac. A 45-year-old man with Meneire-like symptoms underwent contrast-enhanced MRI revealing a mengioma adjacent to the right endolymphatic sac. This was resected through a retrolabyrinthine craniotomy with resolution in patient symptoms.

showing improvement of their symptoms 58% having no change, and 11% with worsening. Of the 74 patients studied, 7 (9%) had symptomatic adverse radiation effects. There was no association between decrease in tumor volume and symptomatic improvement. Trigeminal neuralgia was the most common new symptom after radiosurgery.[10] In another report from the same center, the investigators found that trigeminal neuralgia tended to persist after radiosurgery in petroclival meningiomas despite effective tumor control.[11] In a study by Park and colleagues,[10] measurable hearing was achieved in 99% of patients, and 97% of patients with serviceable hearing preprocedurally had stable or improved hearing after radiosurgery. Unlike in treatment of VSs, no statistical relationship was found between hearing outcomes and radiation dose to the cochlea in stereotactic radiosurgery of meningiomas. A recent multicenter collaboration confirmed this, showing a 93% 5-year progression-free survival and 9% symptomatic neurologic deterioration. This study calculated a 10-year progression-free survival, of 77%.[12]

Epidermoid

Epidermoids are the next most common CPA lesion and represent approximately 6% of such lesions and 1% or all intracranial tumors.[13] In this location they are thought to develop from sequestered epithelial cell rests from the laterally migrating secondary optic and otic capsules or from developing embryonic neurovasculature. They grow slowly through accumulation of keratin and cholesterol from their squamous epithelial lining.[4] Their peak age of occurrence is 40 with no gender predilection. They tend to spread along normal cleavage planes and surround, not displace, cranial nerves and blood vessels.[13] They are benign lesions, although malignant transformation has been reported.[14]

Length of symptoms in cerebellopontine epidermoids tends to be longer than in other tumors of the same area but can present with as wide a variety of posterior fossa dysfunction.[15] Unique to epidermoids, patients can present with recurrent bouts of aseptic meningitis from inflammation induced by keratin debris. On CT scan, these lesions appear almost isodense to spinal fluid with characteristic irregular margins. The signal intensity of these cysts is slightly higher than cerebrospinal fluid (CSF) on T1- and T2-weighted MRI (**Fig. 3**). Diffusion-weighted image sequences differentiate the epidermoid cyst from spinal fluid based on the restricted diffusion signal in the cyst.[6]

Asymptomatic lesions can be followed, but the only definitive treatment of these lesions is gross total resection of the tumor and its capsule, the part of the tumor responsible for its growth. Safe removal of the capsule may be difficult because it can be firmly adherent to the neurovascular structures in the posterior fossa and consequently recurrence is common. Attempts are made to minimize morbidity from cranial nerve dysfunction and in some cases plan to perform serial resections if residual tumor progresses. Retrosigmoid craniotomy serves as the most common surgical approach, although combined approaches, including a subtemporal and transpetrosal approach, may sometimes be used because these tumors may have supratentorial extension (Video 2).

A recent study reports rates of gross total resection of such lesions range from 33% to 88%.[16] In several larger studies in that time period, rates of tumor recurrence have ranged from 7% to 45%. Clinical improvements have been seen in 50% to 100% of the patients. Much as in other surgeries of the CPA, removal of these tumor has risks of facial weakness (0%–23%), worsening of hearing (8%–10%), and swallowing problems (0%–10%). The resection of epidermoids carries a 3% to 8% risk of aseptic meningitis and 0% to 4% of shunted hydrocephalus.[17]

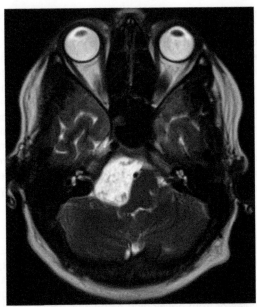

Fig. 3. Epidermoid involving the CPA. A 19-year-old woman with an intracranial epidermoid that involved the right CPA as demonstrated by restricted diffusion on MRI. This was approached through a trasnpetrosal combined retrolabyrinthine posterior fossa and temporal craniotomies for complete resection.

Arachnoid Cyst

Arachnoid cysts compose 1% of all tumors and less than 1% of CPA tumors. Only 7% of all arachnoid cysts are in the CPA and only 15% of which become symptomatic. There is a male predominance overall, but there is a female predominance in cerebellopontine cysts.[18]

These are presumably congenital malformations of the arachnoid and are histologically characterized by a cyst wall made of arachnoid or ependyma and a cystic space filled with CSF or xanthochromic fluid.[4] Their cause is unknown. On CT and MRI they appear almost identical in signal to spinal fluid. They have smooth and rounded edges, displace neurovascular structures, and erode adjacent bony structures.[6] In the CPA they can present with brainstem and cerebellar compression, cranial nerve dysfunction (most commonly CN VIII), mass effect in the posterior fossa resulting in suboccipital headache, tonsillar descent, and syringomyelia.[19] Only 2% of arachnoid cysts have been found to grow.[20] Occasionally, so-called giant arachnoid granulations may be seen as in **Fig. 4**. These too do not enhance with contrast and are T1 isointense.

Asymptomatic arachnoid cysts may be followed clinically because so few of them change. For symptomatic arachnoid cysts, surgery is the only treatment. Options include open surgical resection of all of the cyst walls, open surgical cyst wall fenestration, endoscopic cyst wall fenestration, and cyst shunting or aspiration. The latter 2 procedures are not recommended as first-line treatments because aspiration does not provide durable treatment results and shunts have their own tendency to fail.[19] The preferred approach for open surgery is the retrosigmoid craniotomy. Although series have been small, open surgical resection and fenestration have demonstrated good

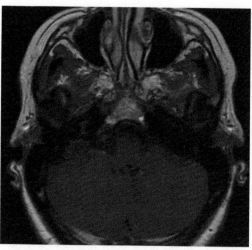

Fig. 4. Giant arachnoid granulation of the CPA. A 51-year-old woman with headaches underwent an MRI that revealed a T1 isointense right CPA lesion and, as seen in this postcontrast image, did not enhance. Given these characteristics, this is most likely a giant arachnoid granulation eroding the internal auditory canal and involving the vestibular aqueduct.

success in treating the condition with improvement in presenting symptoms and an acceptable safety profile.[19] One study did also show that endoscopic fenestration has similar success and safety profile in treatment of posterior fossa arachnoid cysts.[21]

Extension of Intra-axial Posterior Fossa Pathology

Tumors of the brainstem and cerebellum can extend into the CPA where they can mimic more commonly encountered tumors. Brainstem gliomas may extend from the floor or the lateral recesses of the fourth ventricle.[22] Stark and colleagues[23] presented a case of a glioblastoma of the CPA that was resected via a suboccipital approach. There are also several reports of pilocytic astrocytomas originating in the CPA including expansion of the internal acoustic meatus as commonly seen with VSs.[24] Low-grade gliomas may be managed with resection alone, whereas optimal treatment of higher-grade tumors may necessitate radiation, chemotherapy, or both. High-grade, infiltrating tumors may not be amenable to surgical resection.

Choroid plexus papillomas, a tumor derived from the epithelial cells of the choroid plexus, have been reported both extending from the 4th ventricle through the foramen of Luschka and primarily in the CPA. Fourth ventricular tumors and tumors primarily in the CPA tend to present in adults.[25] They compose less than 1% of all intracranial tumors and are benign lesions that can be managed solely with surgery. Less common are more aggressive lesions—so-called atypical papillomas and carcinomas.[13] Overall, 6% of papillomas recur and need repeated surgical intervention.[26] In the pre–MRI era, a series of 12 choroid plexus papillomas of the CPA were resected either through midline approach via the cerebellomedullary fissure or a retromastoid approach. Seven of those patients improved but 2 patients recurred.[25]

Similarly, medulloblastoma, which is classically a pediatric midline cerebellar tumor, can present in adults more laterally and in rare cases in the CPA.[27] These lesions are all World Health Organization (WHO) grade IV and require staging to determine if there are drop metastases elsewhere in the central nervous system. The Goal of treatment is maximal safe resection followed by craniospinal radiation with or without adjuvant chemotherapy (depending on presence of metastases and extent of resection).[13] In the largest series of CPA medulloblastomas, gross total resection through a suboccipital retromastoid craniotomy was achieved in 7 of 14 patients. Eight patients received radiotherapy and 3 received chemotherapy. Within a mean follow-up period of 9 months, 2 patients had symptomatic recurrences that needed further treatment.

Ependymomas, too, can present in the CPA. Intracranially this tumor can develop from cells lining the floor or roof of the fourth ventricle as well as the lateral parts of the medullary velum, which leads to extension into the CPA.[28] Ependymomas may also arise from the spinal cord and filum terminale. Like medulloblastomas they have the potential to seed the spinal fluid. The best outcomes are with gross total resection and radiotherapy.[13] There are several reports of successful resection of CPA ependymomas.[29]

Extension of Extra-axial Pathology

Less commonly, tumors from adjacent non-neural anatomic structures can invade the CPA. Craniopharyngiomas, which arise from residual cells of Rathke pouch, for example, most commonly arise in the suprasellar region and extend cranially.[13] They may extend into the posterior fossa as well, including the CPA. There are, also 2 cases in the literature of craniopharyngiomas arising primarily in the CPA,[30] 1 of which was associated with Gardner syndrome.[31] Both cases were successfully removed via the suboccipital approach. The Goal of treatment is radical resection with the possibility of adjuvant radiotherapy for tumor remnants.[32]

Similarly, chordomas, which are rare tumors arising from the remnants of the primitive notochord, can extend into the CPA.[13] Intracranially they usually extend from the clivus, although there have been several reports of primary intradural chordomas.[33] There is 1 case reported of an intradural chordoma arising in the CPA. This lesion was adherent to the brainstem and cranial nerves and subtotally resected via a subtemporal approach.[34] Outcomes in skull base chordomas tend to be best in those who receive gross total resection and radiotherapy.[35]

Paragangliomas

Lesions affecting the jugular foramen may extend into the CPA. In particular, large glomus jugulare tumors may have a significant CPA component (**Fig. 5**). It is the glomus jugulare subtype that is most likely to involve the CPA. On MRI, these lesions are hypointense on T1, hyperintense on T2, and enhance with gadolinium.

Many centers have moved away from microsurgical resection in favor of stereotactic radiosurgery for such lesions because of the risk of lower cranial nerve dysfunction. Stereotactic radiation therapy is also a primary option for lesions with more limited extension. A newer paradigm for these lesions is dictated by patient symptomatology.[36] When pulsatile tinnitus and conductive hearing loss is bothersome to a patient, a targeted debulking of the middle ear and mastoid component may be undertaken. If indicated based on growth of the remaining lesion, adjuvant radiotherapy may be pursued. Unlike when complete resection is planned, the authors have found preoperative embolization is not needed when only a limited debulking is planned.

Endolymphatic Sac Tumors and Hemangioblastoma

Endolymphatic sac tumors (ELSTs) are rare and most often associated with von Hippel-Landau (VHL) disease, although approximately 20% of cases result from sporadic mutations. Nevoux and colleagues[37] have posited that sporadic tumors

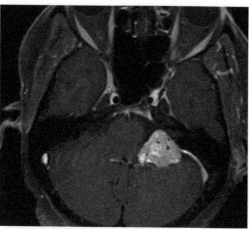

Fig. 5. Glomus tumor involving the CPA. An 80-year-old woman with asymptomatic glomus jugulare, including left CPA component, seen in this enhanced MRI. Patient was referred for low-dose external beam radiation because of tumor extension into the neck.

behave quite differently from those associated with VHL. VHL may affect other organ systems, including cysts throughout the urogenital system, hemangioblastomas of the central nervous system (that may also present in the CPA) and certain malignancies. A majority of patients with VHL inherit this via an autosomal dominant pattern from mutations on chromosome 3.

Pathologically, ELSTs are benign low-grade tumors but may be locally aggressive including erosion into the otic capsule. They are present in 10% of patients with VHL. They may cause progressive hearing loss[38] as well as tinnitus and vertigo. Characteristic imaging findings include T1 hyperintensity with heterogenous enhancement with gadolinium contrast material. CT may also be helpful in demonstrating a destructive lesion centered at the posterior petrous temporal bone in the region of the vestibular aqueduct. Calcifications may be present as well (**Fig. 6**). Histologically, these lesions are characterized as papillary adenomatous lesions and in some cases are classified as adenocarcinomas. Early gross total resection is advocated because of the high risk for recurrence in cases of when a subtotal resection is undertaken. Additionally larger lesions pose increased risk to postoperative facial nerve function.[38] With larger lesions, preoperative embolization may be prudent because these tumors may be supplied by branches of the external carotid or vertebral arteries.[37] In cases where complete surgical resection is not possible or in poor surgical candidates, data suggest a role for adjuvant radiation therapy or primary sterotactic radiotherapy.[38]

Small, less-extensive lesions may be approached from a retrolabyrinthine approach, allowing access to the endolymphatic sac for complete resection of these lesions. This approach also allows for preservation of hearing, as Kim and colleagues[39] demonstrated in maintaining stable pure-tone average in 30 of 31 ears operated via this approach. Depending on a patient's preoperative hearing status, other approaches, including the translabyrinthine route, may be used.

Hemangioblastomas are benign vascular neoplasms that may also be seen in isolation or in association with VHL disease in 25% of cases. They tend to be found in the cerebellum, although their imaging findings on MRI mimic that of VSs (**Fig. 7**), making definitive preoperative diagnosis difficult.[40] When seen, characteristic vascular flow voids may help in making this distinction. Preoperative embolization may be used to

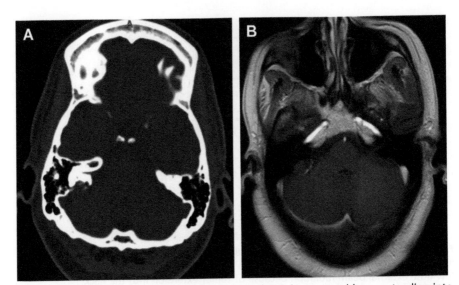

Fig. 6. ELST. A 54-year-old woman with a mass in the right temporal bone extending into the CPA consistent with an ELST. (*A*) Lytic changes in the retrolabyrinthine temporal bone and central calcific spicules are seen on CT. (*B*) T1-enhanced MRI with shows heterogenous enhancement of this lobulated lesion.

facilitate tumor dissection. Although gross total resection is the treatment of choice, radiation may be used for recurrent cases or incomplete resections.

Hemangiopericytomas

Hemangiopericytomas are most often seen supratentorially, but lesions in the CPA have been observed. These lesions are particularly difficult to definitively diagnose because they overlap with meningiomas and solitary fibrous tumors in their clinical

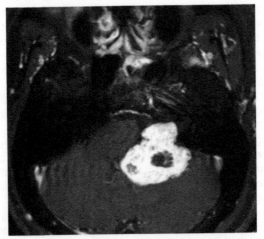

Fig. 7. Hemangioblastoma of the CPA. A 60-year-old man with hemangioblastoma of left CPA underwent subtotal resection via a retrosigmoid craniotomy and postoperative radiation therapy.

and radiologic and pathologic features, although hemangiopericytomas have greater risk for metastatic potential and recurrence.[41] Because of this, these lesions are often treated with adjuvant radiation. **Fig. 8** shows preoperative MRI from a recent patient treated at the authors' institution. She underwent gross total resection of her lesion and was prescribed adjuvant radiation treatment based on final pathology that demonstrated malignant potential.

Lipomas

Although rare, lipomas of the CPA are unique in that accurate preoperative diagnosis on imaging is critical to prevent unnecessary interventions. They account for less than 1% of CPA lesions, and long-term follow-up studies from several institutions suggest very slow if any growth over time.[42,43] Lipomas may involve the CPA and the internal auditory canal and be confused clinically with VSs. Although CPA lipomas may lead to cochleovestibular symptoms, they may often be incidentally discovered in asymptomatic patients. In almost all cases, they tend to be indolent tumors best managed conservatively to minimize patient morbidity. These lesions are hyperintense on T1-weighted imaging, do not enhance with contrast, and lose their signal on fat-suppression sequences.

Intracranial lipomas are thought to be congenital developmental malformations of the meninges rather than true neoplasms. They often display an infiltrative growth pattern along neurovascular structures rather than pushing at the tumor perimeter.[44] This etiology may explain why growth is so rarely observed after diagnosis. The Mayo Clinic recently published their experience in 15 cases over a 20-year period, all but 1 of which was observed with serial imaging.[43] In cases of local mass effect exerting intractable symptoms, operative resection may be offered with the goal of decompression of involved cranial nerves and debulking of the tumor.

Lymphoma

Malignant lymphoma may involve the CPA as a primary intra-axial lymphoma, extension from an extra-axial site, or leptomeningeal lymphoma presenting in the CPA.[45] Accurate diagnosis of lymphoma often requires tissue confirmation and doing so before determining treatment options may prevent significant morbidity to such patients. Although radiology can narrow the differential diagnosis, pathologic biopsy

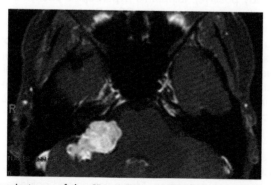

Fig. 8. Hemangiopericytoma of the CPA. A 30-year-old woman with hemangiopericytoma occupying the right CPA as seen on this contrast-enhanced T1 MRI. She underwent preoperative embolization, surgical resection through a suboccipital craniotomy, and postoperative fractionated radiation therapy.

may be required for confirmation. On MRI, lymphoma is most often hypo- or isointense on both T1- and T2-weighted MRI with heterogeneous enhancement. If lymphoma cannot be ruled out on frozen section, it is most prudent to await final pathology findings before proceeding with resection. Radiation therapy is the mainstay treatment of central nervous system lymphoma after a metastatic work-up is completed and so potential surgical morbidities should be avoided.

Metastases

Metastases to the CPA account for less than 1% of CPA tumors. The most common mestatases are from breast, lung, melanoma, thyroid, kidney, and prostate. The clinical history, including a documented or suspected concurrent malignancy along with progressive cranial nerve deficits and bilateral lesions, may aid in diagnosis.

On MRI, these lesions typically are iso-/hypointense on T1-weighted imaging but enhance uniformly with contrast and so may mimic the much more common VS.[46] Lumbar puncture allows for analysis of CSF and so may allow for detection of malignant cells on cytology and hence aid in diagnosis. Eisen and colleagues[47] advocated for this strategy in a series of 7 patients with CPA masses and progressive facial paralysis, 5 of whom had positive malignant cells. Additionally, the determination of whether the malignancy is disseminated in cytologic specimens may help to determine whether surgical resection is appropriate for management. In most cases, resection of only solitary intracranial metastases is considered. Gamma Knife radiation may also be considered for multiple lesions, for leptomeningeal spread, or as an alternative to surgical resection.[48]

Metastatic melanoma is rare but often presents with bilateral lesions, Primary CPA melanoma has also been reported. In the Brackmann and Doherty experience of 6500 CPA tumors reported in 2007, 8 cases of malignant melanoma were noted.[49] Both melanotic and amelanotic melanoma may be seen with subtle differences in imaging characteristics, with amelantoic lesions appearing similar to VSs whereas melanotic lesions are hyperintense on T1-weighted sequences without a decrease in appearance from fat suppression. Definitive pathologic diagnosis is aided by immunohistochemistry, including positive staining for HMB-45 and S-100.

Other Inflammatory Lesions

Dural lesions, such as autoimmune pachymeningitis ANCA (antineutrophil cytoplasmic autoantibody positive), idiopathic hypertrophic pachymeningitis, and other meningeal inflammations, may occur in the CPA. They may present with typical symptoms of CPA lesions as hypertrophied dura compresses cranial nerves. Serologic studies, including autoimmune antibodies, may be useful in the appropriate clinical setting. Infectious etiologies, including Lyme and tuberculosis, should be ruled out. MRI demonstrates dural enhancement with gadolinium in hypertrophic pachymeningitis.[50] Although noncontrast MRI may detect features of dural inflammation, gadolinium is required to assure proper diagnosis of the described patterns.[51] Corticosteroids are the treatment of choice.

SUMMARY

Lesions of the CPA represent 10% of intracranial neoplasms. More than 80% of these are cranial nerve schwannomas. Meningiomas and epidermoids are the next most common followed by a potpourri of other lesions. Focused attention to a patient's clinical history and imaging studies, will often support a particular diagnosis. Because of the variability in how these different pathologies are managed, accurate diagnosis is critical and may require dedicated operative biopsy. Treatment may include observation, microsurgical resection, sterotactic radiation, or multimodality therapy.

SUPPLEMENTARY DATA

Supplementary data related to this article can be found online at http://dx.doi.org/10.1016/j.otc.2015.02.006.

REFERENCES

1. Zúccaro G, Sosa F. Cerebellopontine angle lesions in children. Childs Nerv Syst 2007;23(2):177–83.
2. Batjer HH, Loftus CM, editors. Textbook of neurological surgery: Principles and practice. Philadelphia: Lippincott Williams & Wilkins; 2002.
3. Voss NF, Vrionis FD, Heilman CB, et al. Meningiomas of the cerebellopontine angle. Surg Neurol 2000;53(5):439–47.
4. Springborg JB, Poulsgaard E, Thomsen J. Nonvestibular schwannoma tumors in the cerebellopontine angle: a structured approach and management guidelines. Skull Base 2008;18(4):217–27.
5. Granick MS, Martuza RL, Parker SW, et al. Cerebellopontine angle meningiomas: clinical manifestations and diagnosis. Ann Otol Rhinol Laryngol 1985;94(1 Pt 1): 34–8.
6. Bonneville F, Sarrazin JL, Marsot-Dupuch K, et al. Unusual lesions of the cerebellopontine angle: a segmental approach. Radiographics 2001;21(2):419–38.
7. Thamburaj K, Radhakrishnan VV, Thomas B, et al. Intratumoral microhemorrhages on T2*-weighted gradient-echo imaging helps differentiate vestibular schwannoma from meningioma. AJNR Am J Neuroradiol 2008;29(3):552–7.
8. Coelho DH, Roland JT Jr, Golfinos JG. Posterior fossa meningiomas presenting with Meniere's-like symptoms: case report. Neurosurgery 2008;63(5):E1001 [discussion: E1001].
9. Nicolato A, Foroni R, Pellegrino M, et al. Gamma knife radiosurgery in meningiomas of the posterior fossa. Experience with 62 treated lesions. Minim Invasive Neurosurg 2001;44(04):211–7.
10. Park SH, Kano H, Niranjan A, et al. Stereotactic radiosurgery for cerebellopontine angle meningiomas. J Neurosurg 2013;120(3):708–15.
11. Kano H, Awan NR, Flannery TJ, et al. Stereotactic radiosurgery for patients with trigeminal neuralgia associated with petroclival meningiomas. Stereotact Funct Neurosurg 2011;89(1):17–24.
12. Ding D, Starke RM, Kano H, et al. Gamma knife radiosurgery for cerebellopontine angle meningiomas: a multicenter study. Neurosurgery 2014;75(4):398–408.
13. Greenberg M, editor. Handbook of neurosurgery. 7th edition. New York: Thieme; 2010.
14. Feng R, Gu X, Hu J, et al. Surgical treatment and radiotherapy of epidermoid cyst with malignant transformation in cerebellopontine angle. Int J Clin Exp Med 2014; 7(1):312–5.
15. Mallucci CL, Ward V, Carney AS, et al. Clinical features and outcomes in patients with non-acoustic cerebellopontine angle tumours. J Neurol Neurosurg Psychiatry 1999;66(6):768–71.
16. Gopalakrishnan CV, Ansari KA, Nair S, et al. Long term outcome in surgically treated posterior fossa epidermoids. Clin Neurol Neurosurg 2014;117(0):93–9.

17. Samii M, Tatagiba M, Piquer J, et al. Surgical treatment of epidermoid cysts of the cerebellopontine angle. J Neurosurg 1996;84(1):14–9.
18. Helland CA, Lund-Johansen M, Wester K. Location, sidedness, and sex distribution of intracranial arachnoid cysts in a population-based sample. J Neurosurg 2010;113(5):934–9.
19. Jallo GI, Woo HH, Meshki C, et al. Arachnoid cysts of the cerebellopontine angle: diagnosis and surgery. Neurosurgery 1997;40(1):31–8.
20. Al-Holou WN, Terman S, Kilburg C, et al. Prevalence and natural history of arachnoid cysts in adults. J Neurosurg 2012;118(2):222–31.
21. Gangemi M, Seneca V, Colella G, et al. Endoscopy versus microsurgical cyst excision and shunting for treating intracranial arachnoid cysts. J Neurosurg Pediatr 2011;8(2):158–64.
22. House JL, Burt MR. Primary CNS tumors presenting as cerebellopontine angle tumors. AmJ Otol 1985;(Suppl):147–53.
23. Stark AM, Maslehaty H, Hugo HH, et al. Glioblastoma of the cerebellum and brainstem. J Clin Neurosci 2010;17(10):1248–51.
24. Takada Y, Ohno K, Tamaki M, et al. Cerebellopontine angle pilocytic astrocytoma mimicking acoustic schwannoma. Neuroradiology 1999;41(12):949–50.
25. Talacchi A, De Micheli E, Lombardo C, et al. Choroid plexus papilloma of the cerebellopontine angle: a twelve patient series. Surg Neurol 1999;51(6):621–9.
26. Jeibmann A, Wrede B, Peters O, et al. Malignant progression in choroid plexus papillomas. J Neurosurg Pediatr 2007;107(3):199–202.
27. Jaiswal AK, Mahapatra AK, Sharma MC. Cerebellopointine angle medulloblastoma. J Clin Neurosci 2004;11(1):42–5.
28. Woltman HW, Kernohan JW, Adson AW. Gliomas of the cerebellopontine angle. Proc Staff Meet Mayo Clin 1949;24(3):77–83.
29. Ueyama T, Tamaki N, Kondoh T, et al. Cerebellopontine angle ependymoma with internal auditory canal enlargement and pineal extension—case report&mdash. Neurol Med Chir (Tokyo) 1997;37(10):762–5.
30. Gokalp HZ, Mertol T. Cerebellopontine angle craniopharyngioma. Neurochirurgia (Stuttg) 1990;33(1):20–1.
31. Link MJ, Driscoll CL, Giannini C. Isolated, giant cerebellopontine angle craniopharyngioma in a patient with gardner syndrome: case report. Neurosurgery 2002;51(1):221–6.
32. Elliott RE, Wisoff JH. Successful surgical treatment of craniopharyngioma in very young children. J Neurosurg Pediatr 2009;3(5):397–406.
33. Tashiro T, Fukuda T, Inoue Y, et al. Intradural chordoma: case report and review of the literature. Neuroradiology 1994;36(4):313–5.
34. Mapstone TB, Kaufman B, Ratcheson RA. Intradural chordoma without bone involvement: nuclear magnetic resonance (NMR) appearance. J Neurosurg 1983;59(3):535–7.
35. Samii A, Gerganov VM, Herold C, et al. Chordomas of the skull base: surgical management and outcome. J Neurosurg 2007;107(2):319–24.
36. Miller JP, Semaan M, Einstein D, et al. Staged gamma knife radiosurgery after tailored surgical resection: a novel treatment paradigm for glomus jugulare tumors. Stereotact Funct Neurosurg 2009;87(1):31–6.
37. Nevoux J, Nowak C, Vellin JF, et al. Management of endolymphatic sac tumors: sporadic cases and von Hippel-Lindau disease. Otol Neurotol 2014;35(5):899–904.
38. Carlson ML, Thom JJ, Driscoll CL, et al. Management of primary and recurrent endolymphatic sac tumors. Otol Neurotol 2013;34(5):939–43.

39. Kim HJ, Hagan M, Butman JA, et al. Surgical resection of endolymphatic sac tumors in von Hippel-Lindau disease: findings, results, and indications. Laryngoscope 2013;123(2):477–83.
40. Bush ML, Pritchett C, Packer M, et al. Hemangioblastoma of the cerebellopontine angle. Arch Otolaryngol Head Neck Surg 2010;136(7):734–8.
41. Tashjian VS, Khanlou N, Vinters HV, et al. Hemangiopericytoma of the cerebellopontine angle: a case report and review of the literature. Surg Neurol 2009;72(3): 290–5.
42. Mukherjee P, Street I, Irving RM. Intracranial lipomas affecting the cerebellopontine angle and internal auditory canal: a case series. Otol Neurotol 2011;32(4): 670–5.
43. White JR, Carlson ML, Van Gompel JJ, et al. Lipomas of the cerebellopontine angle and internal auditory canal: primum non nocere. Laryngoscope 2013; 123(6):1531–6.
44. Saunders JE, Kwartler JA, Wolf HK, et al. Lipomas of the internal auditory canal. Laryngoscope 1991;101(10):1031–7.
45. Nishimura T, Uchida Y, Fukuoka M, et al. Cerebellopontine angle lymphoma: a case report and review of the literature. Surg Neurol 1998;50(5):480–5 [discussion: 485–6].
46. Warren FM, Shelton C, Wiggins RH 3rd, et al. Imaging characteristics of metastatic lesions to the cerebellopontine angle. Otol Neurotol 2008;29(6):835–8.
47. Eisen MD, Smith PG, Judy KD, et al. Cerebrospinal fluid cytology to aid the diagnosis of cerebellopontine angle tumors. Otol Neurotol 2006;27(4):553–9.
48. Somaza S, Kondziolka D, Lunsford LD, et al. Stereotactic radiosurgery for cerebral metastatic melanoma. J Neurosurg 1993;79(5):661–6.
49. Brackmann DE, Doherty JK. CPA melanoma: diagnosis and management. Otol Neurotol 2007;28(4):529–37.
50. Kupersmith MJ, Martin V, Heller G, et al. Idiopathic hypertrophic pachymeningitis. Neurology 2004;62(5):686–94.
51. Oghalai JS, Ramirez AL, Hegarty JL, et al. Chronic pachymeningitis presenting as asymmetric sensorineural hearing loss. Otol Neurotol 2004;25(4):616–21.

Petroclival Meningiomas

 CrossMark

Jacob B. Hunter, MD[a],*, Kyle D. Weaver, MD[b],
Reid C. Thompson, MD[b], George B. Wanna, MD[a]

KEYWORDS

- Petroclival • Meningioma • Skull base • Approaches • Outcomes • Complications

KEY POINTS

- Approximately 2% of meningiomas are located in the petroclival region, most commonly encountered in women around the age of 50 years.
- Preoperative imaging includes computed tomography and MRI, while 4-vessel cerebral angiography is commonly obtained.
- Common surgical approaches include retrosigmoid, Kawase, orbitozygomatic, and transpetrosal approaches.
- With the tendency to grow and affect several cranial nerves if observed, general current management trends support subtotal resection with postoperative radiotherapy with 10-year progression-free survival around 80%.
- Complications include cranial nerve deficits, cerebrospinal fluid leakage, hydrocephalus, and brainstem infarctions.

INTRODUCTION

Petroclival meningiomas are intracranial masses with dural attachments to the petroclival synchondrosis, typically near the upper two-thirds of the clivus. Some authors further delineate petroclival meningiomas as those medial to the cranial nerve (CN) foramina V through XI, while others only consider petroclival meningiomas as those medial to the trigeminal nerve (**Fig. 1**).[1–3] With petroclival meningiomas originating near the petroclival suture, given the variety of shapes and sizes, significant neighboring structures can be compromised, including the internal auditory meatus, Meckel cave, cavernous sinus, jugular foramen, parasellar region, foramen magnum, as well as the brainstem, dura, and underlying bone. As such, it is difficult to compare tumor behavior and treatment outcomes between patients and series given the variety of tumor shapes and locations.

Disclosures: None.
[a] Department of Otolaryngology-Head and Neck Surgery, Vanderbilt University Medical Center, 7209 Medical Center East South Tower, 21st Avenue South, Nashville, TN 37232, USA;
[b] Department of Neurological Surgery, Vanderbilt University Medical Center, 1161 21st Avenue South, Rm T-4224 MCN, Nashville, TN 37232, USA
* Corresponding author. Department of Otolaryngology-Head and Neck Surgery, Vanderbilit University Medical Center, 7209 Medical Center East South Tower, 21st Avenue South, Nashville, TN 37232.
E-mail address: jacob.b.hunter@vanderbilt.edu

Otolaryngol Clin N Am 48 (2015) 477–490
http://dx.doi.org/10.1016/j.otc.2015.02.007
0030-6665/15/$ – see front matter © 2015 Elsevier Inc. All rights reserved.

oto.theclinics.com

Abbreviations	
CN	Cranial nerve
CSF	Cerebrospinal fluid
CT	Computed tomography
GTR	Gross-total resection
IAC	Internal auditory canal
KPS	Karnofsky Performance Status
NF	Neurofibromatosis
WHO	World Health Organization

Hallpeau is first credited with describing a petroclival meningioma in a 50-year-old woman in 1874, with most subsequent reports describing patients presenting with motor nerve impairments secondary to tumor compression.[4] Almost 80 years later, in 1953, Castellano and Ruggiero[5] first classified posterior fossa meningiomas, describing the posterior portion of the petrous bone as 1 of 5 possible locations of tumor origination. Since then, further classifications have been described as well as an evolution of treatment strategies. In regards to meningiomas at all locations, the World Health Organization (WHO) classifies 16 different subtypes based on histopathology, categorized into 3 grade designations.[6] Although benign (WHO I) tumors constitute 80% to 90% of all meningiomas, atypical (WHO II) tumors constitute 4.7% to 7.2%, and anaplastic or malignant (WHO III) tumors constitute 1.0% to 2.8%, recurrence and rates of mortality increase as the tumor grade increases.[6,7] What follows is a literature review regarding the presentation, natural history, treatment, and outcomes of petroclival meningiomas.

GENETICS

The neurofibromatosis 2 (NF2) gene on chromosome 22q is the most common genetic alteration in meningiomas, most frequently leading to a nonfunctional merlin protein.[6] Studies show that loss of heterozygosity of chromosome 22 occurs between 40% and

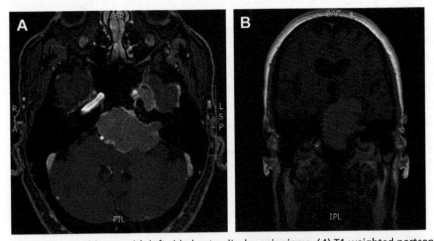

Fig. 1. A 57-year-old man with left-sided petroclival meningioma. (*A*) T1-weighted postcontrast axial image demonstrating tumor within the left IAC and middle fossa, with close association with the left internal carotid artery. (*B*) T1-weighted postcontrast coronal image better demonstrates tumor extension into the IAC.

72% of sporadic meningiomas.[6,7] Nonetheless, NF2 mutations occur equally between meningioma tumor grades.[6,7] Other mutations include 1p deletions, which are co-deleted with chromosome 22q in 67% of meningiomas and are associated with progression and recurrence.[7] Tissue inhibitor of metalloproteinase 3 is another commonly altered gene, found to be hypermethylated in 67% of anaplastic meningiomas, inactivating its tumor suppression activity, compared with only 17% of benign meningiomas.[6] With other epigenetic changes, He and colleagues[8] found that CDKN2 and TP73 gene hypermethylation in meningiomas interacts with the p53 cell cycle regulation, preventing normal cell cycle checkpoint function. Despite these findings, further studies are ongoing to determine factors or profiles that help predict growth and treatment outcomes.

PRESENTATION

Roughly 20% of intracranial masses are meningiomas, 10% of which are located in the posterior fossa, with about 2% of all meningiomas located in the petroclival region.[2,9] Others estimate that petroclival meningiomas account for 0.15% to 0.4% of all intracranial tumors.[1] They are more frequently found in women, ranging in ratios with men from 1.3 to 5.7:1, but generally around 3:1.[10,11] The average age at presentation is between 47.8 and 54.4 years.[10,12]

Studies report a variety of presenting symptoms, including headache, facial numbness, dizziness, and gait disturbances, with many patients also exhibiting facial weakness, hearing impairment, and diplopia. Depending on the report, upwards of 90% of patients in some studies have presented with headaches or gait disturbances, while reports as high as 89% of patients have cranial neuropathies at baseline, with CN V most commonly affected.[1,3]

Initially, poor outcomes were associated with surgical resection; thus, to help compare postoperative outcomes, several studies report performance scores and assessments, including the Karnofsky Performance Status (KPS) score, the Glasgow Outcome Scale, the modified Rankin scale, and the Petroclival Meningioma Impairment Scale. Of the studies that report preoperative KPS scores, scores range from 74.2 to 85.3.[1,12] Not surprisingly, Van Havenbergh and colleagues[13] found a significant inverse correlation between absolute tumor diameters or tumor volumes and KPS scores.

IMAGING

Initially roentgenograms were used to assess skull-base erosion, while cerebral angiography was used to differentiate petroclival meningiomas from intracranial chordomas and brainstem gliomas.[14] The advent of computed tomography (CT) imaging allowed better identification and categorization of all intracranial lesions, with Mayberg and Symon classifying posterior fossa meningiomas based on their site of origin in 1986.[15] On CT imaging, all meningiomas tend to appear slightly hyperdense (70%–75%) to isodense (25%) with broad-based dural attachments.[7] Furthermore, calcification and cyst formation are noted in about 20% of cases, while hyperostosis is seen in 20% to 40%.[7]

In 1987, the first report describing MRI for preoperative evaluation of petroclival meningiomas was published.[16] On MRI, all meningiomas on T1-weighted imaging appear slightly hypointense to isointense, while variably isointense to hyperintense on T2-weighted imaging (**Fig. 2**).[7] In addition, several imaging characteristics are associated with meningiomas, such as peritumoral edema and a "dural tail," the latter of which occurs in 35% to 80% of tumors, best appreciated with the administration of gadolinium (**Fig. 3**).[7] Many studies have reported on MRI in predicting tumor resectability, with edema on T2-weighted imaging suggesting brainstem adherence or invasion, or loss

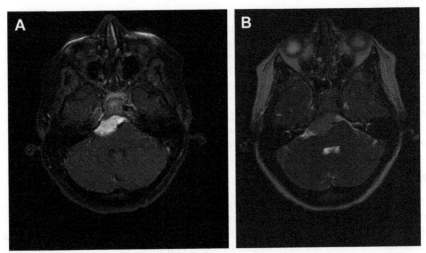

Fig. 2. A 35-year-old woman with right-sided petroclival meningioma. Note the difference in intensity between images. (*A*) T1-weighted postcontrast axial image. (*B*) T2-weighted axial image.

of an arachnoid plane on T1-weighted or T2-weighted imaging indicating pial invasion, findings which would suggest a more difficult resection (**Fig. 4**).[1,9,17]

In addition to preoperative CT and MRI, many groups still use preoperative 4-vessel cerebral angiography to assess the intracranial vasculature. In one of the largest studies to date, Natarajan and colleagues[9] obtained preoperative cerebral angiography on all patients, embolizing 61%. However, most groups will only obtain angiography if the cavernous sinus and the carotid or basilar arteries are involved, and thus, assess if preoperative embolization may facilitate surgical resection (**Fig. 5**).[3,18]

NATURAL HISTORY

The risks, benefits, and alternatives of treating petroclival meningiomas must be weighed against their natural history. Van Havenbergh and colleagues[13] retrospectively reviewed 21 patients with petroclival meningiomas who underwent no treatment for a minimum of 4 years, and an average of almost 7 years. They found that 76% of tumors demonstrated growth on imaging, with 50% of the original asymptomatic patients exhibiting at least one CN deficit, and 20% of those patients with at least one CN deficit developing additional CN involvement.[13] Furthermore, by using either CT or MRI to determine the tumor-equivalent diameter and tumor volume, they found that the overall tumor diameter and tumor volume growth rates were 0.81 mm/y and 0.81 cm³/y, respectively.[13] These growth rates pale in comparison with a previous study reviewing the postoperative courses of 38 patients who underwent subtotal resection of petroclival meningiomas without further treatment, reporting tumor diameter and volume growth rates of 3.7 mm/y and 4.94 cm³/y, respectively.[19] Despite the different growth rates, without intervention, petroclival meningiomas are expected to grow.

TREATMENT

With the propensity for patients with petroclival meningiomas to present with significant complaints and the tendency for the tumors to grow, there are many studies

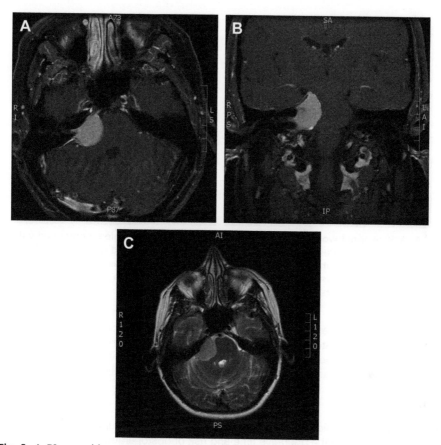

Fig. 3. A 50-year-old woman with a right-sided petroclival meningioma presented with asymmetric hearing loss over the previous 4 to 5 years, as well as tinnitus, and intermittent sharp pain in her right V3 distribution. (*A*) T1-weighted postcontrast axial image demonstrates the dural tail, a feature commonly seen in meningiomas, aiding to differentiate the lesion from a vestibular schwannoma. (*B*) T1-weighted postcontrast coronal image outlines its lateral extension within the right IAC. (*C*) T2-weighted axial imaging.

discussing the variety of treatment options. Although initial reports demonstrated significant morbidity and mortality, with the advent of microsurgical techniques as well as radiotherapy, either modality alone, or together, has greatly reduced the morbidity and mortality in treating these lesions. **Table 1** summarizes all studies reporting at least 50 cases of petroclival meningiomas with surgical intervention.

SURGERY

Given the initial poor outcomes following petroclival meningioma resections, many groups have investigated many different skull-base approaches to best remove these lesions, concurrently minimizing significant complications.

APPROACHES

Many groups have discussed the advantages and disadvantages of surgical approaches with the general theme that the best surgical approach is dictated by

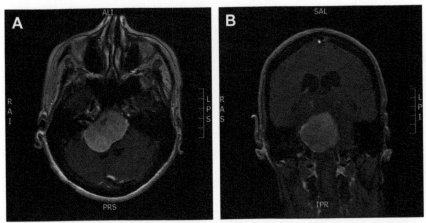

Fig. 4. A 60-year-old woman with a right-sided petroclival meningioma presented with a 1-year history of progressive quadriparesis, difficulty speaking, and difficulty swallowing. (*A*) T1-weighted postcontrast axial image demonstrates a fine arachnoid plane between the tumor and brainstem, likely indicating no pial invasion in that region. (*B*) T1-weighted postcontrast coronal image.

the tumor's location, extent of planned resection, surgeon experience and comfort, and patient's age, anatomy, hearing, and neurologic status. Furthermore, several authors have created algorithms based on tumor locations and CN deficits to determine the best approaches as well as models predicting tumor resectability.[1,14,20]

RETROSIGMOID

The retrosigmoid craniotomy provides access to the petrosal surface of the temporal bone, while reducing the operative time and risk of postoperative cerebrospinal fluid (CSF) leak.[1,17,18,20,21] In patients with serviceable hearing, the approach also provides

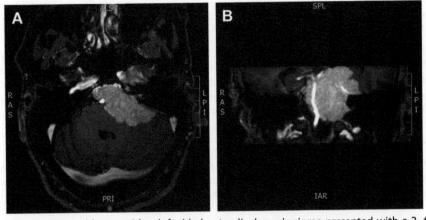

Fig. 5. A 65-year-old man with a left-sided petroclival meningioma presented with a 2- to 3-month history of left-sided facial numbness. (*A*) T1-weighted postcontrast axial image shows the basilar artery almost surrounded by tumor in 270°. (*B*) T1-weighted postcontrast coronal image better highlights the basilar artery in relation to tumor.

a wider angle to infratentorial lesions as compared with the retrolabyrinthine approach. Compared with the Kawase approach, the retrosigmoid approach has been shown to provide larger brainstem and clival working areas.[20] Others use the approach when venous drainage prevents posterior petrosal access.[1] However, the retrosigmoid approach requires significant cerebellar retraction, limiting exposure to the ventral brainstem and entire clivus as well as placing significant risk to the trochlear nerve if the tumor has significant supratentorial extension.[2,18]

KAWASE

First described to access aneurysms of the basilar artery, the Kawase approach accesses skull-base lesions from a middle fossa, or subtemporal, craniotomy.[22] It is limited by the petrous ridge medially, the greater superficial petrosal nerve laterally, the internal auditory canal (IAC) posteriorly, and the mandibular nerve anteriorly, with some groups suggesting it is most appropriate for tumors medial to the IAC with minimal or no posterior fossa involvement.[20]

FRONTOTEMPORAL ORBITOZYGOMATIC

Various authors report on the orbitozygomatic approach, which can be used to access tumors above the tentorial notch, such as those in the suprasellar, parasellar, and retrosellar regions, as well as lesions located at the petrous apex, cavernous sinus, and as far anterior as the orbit.[2,20]

LATERAL SKULL-BASE/TRANSPETROSAL APPROACHES

Many reports support the advantages of petrous bone excision through lateral skull-base approaches, including decreased brain retraction and operative distance, as well as improved visualization and illumination.[1,23] With a variety of descriptions, transpetrosal approaches have many titles and names. Xu and colleagues[20] classify all posterior transpetrosal approaches as variations of the basic mastoidectomy, which include retrolabyrinthine, translabyrinthine, and transcochlear, the latter 2 as options in patients with nonserviceable hearing. Some authors characterize resection of the presigmoid retrolabyrinthine petrous bone as a posterior petrosal approach, which is recommended for patients with serviceable hearing with lesions extending below the internal auditory meatus.[1] Although the translabyrinthine approach provides early identification and minimal manipulation of the facial nerve, the transcochlear approach allows maximal exposure to the ventral brainstem, requiring facial nerve rerouting. Tumors located in the upper two-thirds of the clivus, or medial or superior to the internal auditory meatus, can be approached through an anterior transpetrosal, transtentorial approach, through a subtemporal craniotomy.[12] Others advocate combined approaches for tumors extending across midline, or into the cavernous sinus, such as a combined anterior and posterior petrosal approach. However, combined approaches increase the risk of postoperative CSF leakage, facial or cochleovestibular nerve injury, and injury to the vein of Labbe, while requiring temporal lobe retraction and increasing the operative time.[1,2,20]

SURGICAL RESECTION

Maximizing tumor resection while minimizing postoperative complications is the challenge of all tumor surgery. To help facilitate comparison between cases and series, several grading scales have been developed in an attempt to categorize the amount of tumor that was resected. The most commonly used scale is the Simpson grading

Table 1
Chronologic listing of all petroclival meningioma surgical case series of 50 patients or more

Study, year	N	M:F Ratio	Avg. Age	MTV	Mean Preoperative KPS	Most Common Presenting Symptom	GTR (%)	Mean F/U (mo)	Mortality (%)	CN Deficits (%)	Complications (%)	Recurrence (%)	Mean Time to Recurrence (mo)
Couldwell et al,[3] 1996	109	1:1.7	51.0			Gait disturbance/headache (90%)	69.0		3.7	33.0	32.1	13.0	73.2
Sekhar et al,[17] 1996	75	1:2.4											
Carvalho,[35] 2000	70	1:2.3	49.0					52.8					
Roberti et al,[26] 2001	110				82	Headache 50%	45.0		1.0		89.6		
Little et al,[18] 2005	137	1:2.6	53.0			55% (31% overall had CN V weakness)	40.0	8.3	0.8	22.6	16.7	17.6	
Natarajan et al,[9] 2007	150	1:4.2	51.0	3.44 cm (TED)	78		32.0	101.6		20.3	22.0	4.7	72.0

Study													
Li et al,[24] 2010	57	1:3.1	50.5				58.0			67.0	42.0	12.3	42.0
Seifert,[11] 2010	148	1:1.3					37.0						
Nanda et al,[2] 2011	50	1:2.6	55.0				28.0	22.1		44.0		19.0	84.0
Chen,[36] 2011	82		53.2		3.64 cm³	Headache and facial hypothesia 53.7%	56.1		2.4		24.0		
Li et al,[12] 2013	259	1:2.7	47.8	74.2	4.54 cm³	Headache 31.7%	52.5	55.3		28.2		4.5	40.7
Almefty et al,[1] 2014	64	1:3	49.0	85.3	3.55 (max. tumor d)	Facial numbness and hearing loss 37.5%	64.0	70.6	1.6	39.0			
Morisako et al,[10] 2015	60	1:5.7	54.4			106							

Several studies included the same patients more than once and were excluded.
Abbreviations: CN, cranial nerve; GTR, gross-total resection; MTV, mean tumor volume; TED, tumor equivalent diameter.
Data from Refs. [1–3,9–12,17,18,24,26,35,36]

scale, categorizing tumor resection into 4 groups, while others use the modified Shinshu grading scale, also known as the Okudesa-Kobayashi scale, delineating 7 categories.[1] Gross-total resection (GTR), which is defined as complete macroscopic tumor removal with no radiographic evidence of lesions on postoperative imaging, is scored as I on both the Simpson and the Kobayashi grading scales, with the grades increasing as more tumor remains. Others report only the percentage of remaining tumor based on postoperative imaging. The prevailing hypothesis is that the more residual tumor that remains, the more likely the tumor will recur, whereas the more tumor that is removed, the more likely patients will have postoperative CN deficits or significant complications.

In addition, many groups report on tumor involvement within the cavernous sinus or Meckel cave. In the largest published petroclival meningioma series to date, out of China, Li and colleagues[12] reported on 259 patients, with 116 (73.4%) tumors within the cavernous sinus or Meckel cave completely removed. Given the important surrounding structures, many resections are limited by the involvement of CNs, brainstem or vessels, tumor size or firm consistency, extensive regional involvement, disappearance of the dissection plane, and medical comorbidities.[1,2,12]

With the important surrounding anatomy, and by using operative notes and postoperative imaging, studies report a large range of percentages for complete microscopic removal. In series reviewing greater than 50 cases, GTR percentages range from 28.0% to 69.0%, while in smaller studies, percentages as low as 20%, and as great as 85%, have been reported.[1–3] Many studies also describe the recurrence rate based on the amount of tumor resected. Following GTR, recurrence rates range from 0.7% to 9.8%.[1,12] Not surprisingly, most studies report greater recurrence rates when residual tumor remains, ranging from 5% to 60%.[3,9] Nonetheless, Almefty and colleagues[1] reported on 4 of 13 patients, who were thought to have the entire tumor removed, develop recurrences. Overall, in reviewing those same studies, recurrence rates range from 4.5% to 21.8% after combining resections of all types.[1,12] When individual studies compare recurrence rates following GTRs versus subtotal resection, results have been conflicting.[1,3,18] Natarajan and colleagues[9] found 4% of patients with GTR and 5% of patients with incomplete resection had tumor recurrence, suggesting the extent of resection had no bearing on tumor recurrence. However, the median time to recurrence in patients with GTRs is generally twice as long as compared with patients with subtotal resections, sometimes as long as 168 months following GTRs.[1]

With a range of recurrence rates, several studies have investigated if certain factors could predict recurrence. Variables that have shown correlation to higher recurrence rates include tumor location; tumor size larger than 5 cm; previous treatment; ability to infiltrate bone, muscle, nerve, and vessels; histopathologic grade; irregular shaped tumors; lower extent of resection; and presence of contrast enhancement on postoperative imaging.[2,12]

Given the intricate skull-base anatomy, petroclival meningiomas were first considered inoperable.[14] Before 1970, of all published cases, only 10 of 26 patients survived surgery for tumor extirpation, only one of which had total resection.[14] Fortunately, the mortality has currently decreased to 0.8% to 3.2% in the immediate postoperative period.[3,18] Natarajan and colleagues[9] reported progression-free survival rates, with 3-, 5-, and 10-year progression-free survival rates of all patients to be 98.7%, 92.1%, and 81.9%, respectively. If the patients with GTR were not included in the same calculations, the same progression-free survival rates decrease to 96%, 91.7%, and 79.5%, respectively.[9] In further analyzing those patients with residual tumor who underwent radiosurgery or radiotherapy, there was no significant difference in the progression-free survival of patients who had residual tumors who did not undergo radiosurgery or radiotherapy as compared with those who did.[9]

COMPLICATIONS

In addition to recurrence and mortality, complications including CN deficits, CSF leaks, and brainstem infarctions are commonly reported. Furthermore, many studies also analyze various preoperative and perioperative variables in an attempt to predict postoperative complications.

In regards to CN deficits, the largest series report postoperative deficits ranging from 20.3% to 67%.[9,24] However, the CNs affected postoperatively are not necessarily the ones that were weak preoperatively. Almefty and colleagues[1] demonstrated that CNs V and VIII were most likely to improve following surgery, while CN VI was most likely to be permanently injured. Similarly, Natarajan and colleagues[9] reported that CN VI was most frequently permanently injured, leading to diplopia, the most common long-term disability in their review, affecting 72% of patients. In the largest study to date, comprising 259 patients with petroclival meningiomas, CN III was most commonly injured postoperatively.[12] Still other studies report that CN VII is the most frequently injured postoperatively as well as CN V.[18,24]

Although one might expect more cranial neuropathies with more extensive resections, Almefty and colleagues[1] reported in their series that more complete resections led to fewer CN deficits. Nonetheless, Little and colleagues[18] showed that preoperative CN function, tumor adherence to neurovascular structures, fibrous tumor consistency, and prior resections were significantly associated with postoperative CN deficits, some of the same factors that also predict tumor recurrence. Looking at all complications, Sekhar and colleagues[25] found that male patients, tumors larger than 2.5 cm, tumor blood supply from the basilar artery, brainstem edema, vascular encasement, and diminished KPS scores were significant negative predictors of postoperative complications.

Of interest, one study discussed a specific case within their series that changed their surgical philosophy that led to less aggressive resections. Comparing resection percentages, Little and colleagues[18] found no significant differences in their rates of gross-total, near-total, and subtotal resections before and after their surgical adjustment. However, they noted significantly more CN deficits, with a trend for greater postoperative paresis/ataxia in the more aggressive earlier group.[18] Generally speaking, most groups report aggressively resect cavernous sinus disease if the patient is asymptomatic preoperatively, while leaving residual disease for either observation or postoperative radiosurgery if the patient is symptomatic.[18]

Other complications include CSF leaks, hydrocephalus, hematomas, and brainstem infarctions. With no clear guidelines on what and how to report complications, studies have complication rates, including CN deficits, ranging from 16.7% to 89.6%.[18,26] Most, but not all studies report that CSF leaks, aside from CN deficits, are the second most frequently encountered complication, ranging from 2% to 17%.[2,9] Nanda and colleagues[2] reported the risk of pseudomeningoceles range from 15% to 28%, while in regards to hydrocephalus, which requires placement of ventriculoperitoneal shunts, rates are generally reported to be around 2%.[9,18] Brainstem or brain infarction rates range from 0.8% to 14.7%.[3,9,12] Other commonly reported complications include intracranial infections, tracheostomy rates, symptomatic cerebral edema, brainstem, cerebellar, and abdominal fat graft site hematomas, as well as aspiration pneumonia, pulmonary embolisms, and seizures.[1,3,9,12,18]

RADIATION

Stereotactic radiotherapy and radiosurgery were initially thought to have little influence with meningiomas before 1970, until early studies with all meningiomas demonstrated reduced rates of local recurrence with postoperative radiotherapy.[14] Sekhar and Schramm[16] first suggested postoperative radiotherapy in partially resected petroclival meningiomas in 1987, the same year Barbaro and colleagues[27] reported on patient outcomes in patients with subtotally resected meningiomas in all locations treated with postoperative radiotherapy. Barbaro and colleagues[27] found that the recurrence rate in patients with subtotal resections with and without postoperative radiotherapy was 32% and 60%, respectively, with a significantly longer time period until recurrence development, 125 and 66 months, with and without postoperative radiotherapy. Given these results, the role of radiation in patients with GTRs, as well as subtotal resections was further investigated.

Initial primary radiosurgery studies reported tumor control rates, as defined by no further growth on serial imaging, of 100%, although follow-up periods ranged from 34 to 56 months on average.[28,29] Flannery and colleagues[30] reported on 168 patients with petroclival meningiomas treated with radiosurgery, and although their median follow-up was 64 months with unclear tumor growth definitions, they concluded that radiosurgery prevented initial or further resection in 98% of patients. These same patients were later included in a larger multicenter study consisting of 254 patients with petroclival meningiomas treated with Gamma Knife radiosurgery, with tumor control rates of 93% and 84% at 5 and 10 years, respectively.[31] With reports of CN complications with radiosurgery ranging between 5% and 9.4%, the role of microsurgery and its substantial risks were debated.[12,20,28] Furthermore, with Rowe and colleagues[32] reporting no increased risk of malignancy following radiosurgery for various intracranial pathologic abnormalities in 4877 patients having been followed for 29,916 patient-years, many began entertaining the idea of deficit-free tumor resection, with postoperative radiation for any residual tumor.

However, controversy remains. Starke and colleagues[33] retrospectively reviewed 152 posterior fossa meningiomas and found that radiographic progression-free survival at 3, 5, and 10 years was 98%, 96%, and 78%, respectively, consistent with the rates reported by Natarajan and colleagues[9] following surgery, 98.7%, 92.1%, and 81.9%, respectively.[33] In regards to complications, Mathiesen and colleagues[34] reviewed 45 patients with meningiomas at all locations, treated with fractionated radiotherapy, and found 56% of patients had complications requiring hospitalization or a major change in lifestyle, which included fatigue, feelings of intellectual weakness, and motor deficits. They further added that with some patients demonstrating evidence of recurrence as late as 17 years following treatment, most studies lack the necessary follow-up to make conclusions on the safety of radiation.[34] With ischemic brainstem lesions and CN deficits arising 12 to 18 months following treatment, other groups emphasize that not all complications are immediate, additionally raising the concern that approximately 8% of tumors will continue to grow following radiosurgery.[2] Nevertheless, most experts think that petroclival meningiomas should be resected as much as possible while ensuring the integrity of the CNs, radiating any tumor in patients unfit for surgery or with complicated recurrences.[1,14]

SUMMARY

Petroclival meningiomas account for approximately 2% of intracranial meningiomas, most commonly presenting in women at almost a 3:1 ratio around 50 years of age, with headache and gait disturbances as the most common presenting signs. With the natural tendency to grow and affect other CNs, treatment options include surgery and radiation. Given initial surgical outcomes studies demonstrating significant morbidity and mortality, as well as the development of radiotherapy, current management trends support subtotal resection plus or minus postoperative radiotherapy, with approximately 80% 10-year progression-free survival rates.

REFERENCES

1. Almefty R, Dunn IF, Pravdenkova S, et al. True petroclival meningiomas: results of surgical management. J Neurosurg 2014;120(1):40–51.
2. Nanda A, Javalkar V, Banerjee AD. Petroclival meningiomas: study on outcomes, complications and recurrence rates. J Neurosurg 2011;114(5):1268–77.
3. Couldwell WT, Fukushima T, Giannotta SL, et al. Petroclival meningiomas: surgical experience in 109 cases. J Neurosurg 1996;84(1):20–8.
4. Cushing H. Meningiomas: their classification, regional behaviour, life history, and surgical end results. New York: Hafner Pub. Co; 1962.
5. Castellano F, Ruggiero G. Meningiomas of the posterior fossa. Acta Radiol Suppl 1953;104:1–177.
6. Mawrin C, Perry A. Pathological classification and molecular genetics of meningiomas. J Neurooncol 2010;99(3):379–91.
7. Campbell BA, Jhamb A, Maguire JA, et al. Meningiomas in 2009: controversies and future challenges. Am J Clin Oncol 2009;32(1):73–85.
8. He S, Pham MH, Pease M, et al. A review of epigenetic and gene expression alterations associated with intracranial meningiomas. Neurosurg Focus 2013;35(6):E5.
9. Natarajan SK, Sekhar LN, Schessel D, et al. Petroclival meningiomas: multimodality treatment and outcomes at long-term follow-up. Neurosurgery 2007;60(6): 965–79 [discussion: 979–81].
10. Morisako H, Goto T, Ohata K. Petroclival meningiomas resected via a combined transpetrosal approach: surgical outcomes in 60 cases and a new scoring system for clinical evaluation. J Neurosurg 2015;122(2):373–80.
11. Seifert V. Clinical management of petroclival meningiomas and the eternal quest for preservation of quality of life: personal experiences over a period of 20 years. Acta Neurochir 2010;152(7):1099–116.
12. Li D, Hao SY, Wang L, et al. Surgical management and outcomes of petroclival meningiomas: a single-center case series of 259 patients. Acta Neurochir 2013;155(8):1367–83.
13. Van Havenbergh T, Carvalho G, Tatagiba M, et al. Natural history of petroclival meningiomas. Neurosurgery 2003;52(1):55–62 [discussion: 62–4].
14. Maurer AJ, Safavi-Abbasi S, Cheema AA, et al. Management of petroclival meningiomas: a review of the development of current therapy. J Neurol Surg B Skull Base 2014;75(5):358–67.
15. Mayberg MR, Symon L. Meningiomas of the clivus and apical petrous bone. Report of 35 cases. J Neurosurg 1986;65(2):160–7.
16. Sekhar LN, Schramm VL. Tumors of the cranial base: diagnosis and treatment. Mount Kisco (NY): Futura Pub. Co; 1987.
17. Sekhar LN, Wright DC, Richardson R, et al. Petroclival and foramen magnum meningiomas: surgical approaches and pitfalls. J Neurooncol 1996;29(3): 249–59.
18. Little KM, Friedman AH, Sampson JH, et al. Surgical management of petroclival meningiomas: defining resection goals based on risk of neurological morbidity

and tumor recurrence rates in 137 patients. Neurosurgery 2005;56(3):546–59 [discussion: 546–59].

19. Jung HW, Yoo H, Paek SH, et al. Long-term outcome and growth rate of subtotally resected petroclival meningiomas: experience with 38 cases. Neurosurgery 2000;46(3):567–74 [discussion: 574–5].

20. Xu F, Karampelas I, Megerian CA, et al. Petroclival meningiomas: an update on surgical approaches, decision making, and treatment results. Neurosurg Focus 2013;35(6):E11.

21. Goel A, Muzumdar D. Conventional posterior fossa approach for surgery on petroclival meningiomas: a report on an experience with 28 cases. Surg Neurol 2004;62(4):332–8 [discussion: 338–40].

22. Kawase T, Toya S, Shiobara R, et al. Transpetrosal approach for aneurysms of the lower basilar artery. J Neurosurg 1985;63(6):857–61.

23. Erkmen K, Pravdenkova S, Al-Mefty O. Surgical management of petroclival meningiomas: factors determining the choice of approach. Neurosurg Focus 2005;19(2):E7.

24. Li PL, Mao Y, Zhu W, et al. Surgical strategies for petroclival meningioma in 57 patients. Chin Med J 2010;123(20):2865–73.

25. Sekhar LN, Jannetta PJ, Burkhart LE, et al. Meningiomas involving the clivus: a six-year experience with 41 patients. Neurosurgery 1990;27(5):764–81 [discussion: 781].

26. Roberti F, Sekhar LN, Kalavakonda C, et al. Posterior fossa meningiomas: surgical experience in 161 cases. Surg Neurol 2001;56(1):8–20 [discussion: 20–1].

27. Barbaro NM, Gutin PH, Wilson CB, et al. Radiation therapy in the treatment of partially resected meningiomas. Neurosurgery 1987;20(4):525–8.

28. Roche PH, Pellet W, Fuentes S, et al. Gamma knife radiosurgical management of petroclival meningiomas results and indications. Acta Neurochir 2003;145(10): 883–8 [discussion: 888].

29. Subach BR, Lunsford LD, Kondziolka D, et al. Management of petroclival meningiomas by stereotactic radiosurgery. Neurosurgery 1998;42(3):437–43 [discussion: 443–5].

30. Flannery TJ, Kano H, Lunsford LD, et al. Long-term control of petroclival meningiomas through radiosurgery. J Neurosurg 2010;112(5):957–64.

31. Starke R, Kano H, Ding D, et al. Stereotactic radiosurgery of petroclival meningiomas: a multicenter study. J Neurooncol 2014;119(1):169–76.

32. Rowe J, Grainger A, Walton L, et al. Risk of malignancy after gamma knife stereotactic radiosurgery. Neurosurgery 2007;60(1):60–5 [discussion: 65–6].

33. Starke RM, Nguyen JH, Rainey J, et al. Gamma Knife surgery of meningiomas located in the posterior fossa: factors predictive of outcome and remission. J Neurosurg 2011;114(5):1399–409.

34. Mathiesen T, Kihlstrom L, Karlsson B, et al. Potential complications following radiotherapy for meningiomas. Surg Neurol 2003;60(3):193–8 [discussion: 199–200].

35. Carvalho GA, Matthies C, Tatagiba M, et al. Impact of computed tomographic and magnetic resonance imaging findings on surgical outcome in petroclival meningiomas. Neurosurgery 2000;47(6):1287–94 [discussion:1294–85].

36. Chen LF, Yu ZG, Bu B, et al. The retrosigmoid approach to petroclival meningioma surgery. J Clin Neurosci 2011;18(12):1656–61.

Primary Tumors of the Facial Nerve

Theodore R. McRackan, MD[a], Eric P. Wilkinson, MD[a], Alejandro Rivas, MD[b],*

KEYWORDS

- Facial nerve tumors • Facial nerve schwannoma • Facial nerve neuroma
- Geniculate ganglion hemangioma • Facial nerve vascular malformation
- Glomus facialis • Facial nerve paraganglioma • Facial nerve granular cell tumor

KEY POINTS

- Facial nerve schwannomas are the most common primary tumor of the facial nerve and represent a difficult treatment paradigm.
- There is significant debate over optimal treatment of facial nerve schwannomas with observation, decompression, debulking, resection with facial nerve grafting, and radiosurgery all supported in the literature.
- Geniculate ganglion hemangiomas often present with facial nerve paralysis out of proportion to lesion size on imaging.
- Treatment of geniculate ganglion hemangiomas has changed over time with earlier surgical resection playing a more modern role.

INTRODUCTION

Primary tumors of the facial nerve (FN) are rare with FN schwannomas (FNSs) being the most common of these lesions. Other less frequent tumors include glomus facialis, geniculate ganglion hemangiomas (GGHs), and granular cell tumors. Diagnosis of these lesions can be difficult given the intimate anatomic relationship of these tumors with other structures of the lateral skull base. Treatment is also challenging because the risk of FN injury is high with surgical intervention. Also, given the scarcity of these lesions, it is difficult to develop a clear consensus with regard to treatment. This article discusses the pathophysiology, symptomology, diagnosis, and treatment of these tumors.

FACIAL NERVE SCHWANNOMAS

FNS represents one of the more difficult treatment paradigms in neurotology. These tumors are so rare that determining a true incidence in the general population is

Disclosures: None.
[a] House Ear Clinic, 2100 W 3rd St #111, Los Angeles, CA 90057, USA; [b] Vanderbilt University Medical Center, 7209 Medical Center East-South Tower, 1215 21st Avenue South, Nashville, TN 37232, USA
* Corresponding author.
E-mail address: alejandro.rivas@Vanderbilt.Edu

Otolaryngol Clin N Am 48 (2015) 491–500
http://dx.doi.org/10.1016/j.otc.2015.02.008
0030-6665/15/$ – see front matter © 2015 Elsevier Inc. All rights reserved.

oto.theclinics.com

difficult. Saito and Baxter[1] found 5 (0.83%) incidental FNS in 600 temporal bone specimens representing the best current estimation. However, this collection is not representative of the general population and the actual incidence of FNS remains relatively unknown. This low case prevalence has made development of a uniform treatment algorithm challenging.

Presentation

The presenting symptoms of FNS vary based on tumor size and location. In patients ultimately diagnosed with FNS, hearing loss has been reported in 33% to 78.6%, tinnitus in 7% to 51.8%, and vertigo in 46%.[2–4] Specifically with regard to FN function, 50% to 60% have some history of FN paralysis with approximately 20% of symptoms being transient.[2]

Diagnosis

The patient's physical examination is typically normal with a few exceptions. A thorough FN examination is important to identify any paralysis, twitching, or subtle abnormalities. The otologic examination is typically normal unless the tympanic or mastoid segment is largely involved revealing either a retrotympanic or external auditory canal mass (**Fig. 1**).[5] In such situations tuning fork examination can reveal a conductive loss

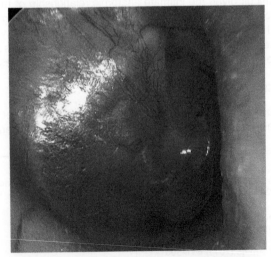

Fig. 1. Otoscopic examination. Facial nerve schwannoma touching the tympanic membrane, occupying the upper two-thirds of the drum.

on the involved side. Similarly, when there is a significant sensorineural hearing loss from an FNS of the internal auditory canal (IAC)/cerebellopontine angle (CPA), the Weber can lateralize to the uninvolved side.

The patient's collective symptoms typically lead to imaging, which is the main diagnostic test for FNS. MRI and computed tomography (CT) can be helpful in diagnosing these lesions. Thin-sectioned MRI with gadolinium can positively identify an enhancing lesion along the FN. When segments proximal and distal to the Geniculate ganglion (GG) are involved, the typical "hourglass" appearance can be observed on the MRI **(Fig. 2)**. However, differentiating FNS from vestibular schwannomas (VS) can be difficult, if not impossible, when only segments proximal to the labyrinthine portion are involved. Likewise, if only the GG, tympanic, and/or vertical segments of the FN are involved, diagnosis can be difficult because these segments can also enhance under normal physiologic conditions. CT can complement MRI in looking at changes to the bony architecture surrounding the FN in the tympanic and mastoid segment, typically showing an enlarged fallopian canal compared with the contralateral side **(Fig. 3)**.

FNS can occur at any point along the FN. The most commonly involved segment is the GG (60%–66%) followed by the tympanic (53%) and labyrinthine segments (50.6%–60%).[3,4] Most tumors involve more than one segment.[2–4,6–10] Skip lesions can be seen on MRI when normal FN exists between involved segments. This has been described as "beads on a string" and has been reported to occur in 20% of cases.[4,11]

Like their vestibular counterparts, FNS arise from the Schwann cells and are arranged in an Antoni A, Antoni B, or combined histologic pattern.[1,12] There has been no described correlation between histologic pattern and tumor behavior.

Treatment

Determining the optimal treatment of an individual patient with an FNS is difficult. The overall goal of FNS treatment is preservation of FN function for the longest duration

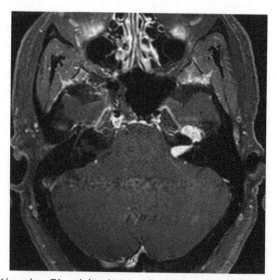

Fig. 2. Classic MRI imaging. T1-weighted MRI with contrast, axial view, showing typical hourglass enhancing appearance of facial nerve schwannoma. Notice enlargement of IAC segment, geniculate ganglion, and greater superficial petrosal nerve, with narrow point at the labyrinthine segment.

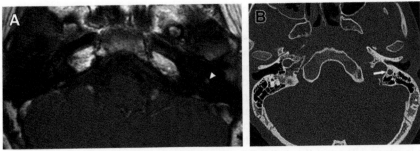

Fig. 3. Facial nerve schwannoma in the mastoid segment. (A) T1-weighted MRI with contrast, axial view, showing light enhancement of the vertical segment (*arrowhead*), which could be confused with physiologic enhancement. (B) CT showing obvious enlargement of fallopian canal (*arrow*), compared with the contralateral side.

possible assuming other symptoms do not require intervention. Examination of the literature shows a wide variety of treatment methods. These range from conservative management with periodic imaging, decompression, tumor debulking or stripping, and resection with FN graft if possible.

One of the main difficulties in diagnosing and treating FNS is that many are initially thought to be VS until the tumor is exposed in surgery. This is particularly true when only the IAC and CPA are involved with tumor. Rates of FNS thought preoperatively to be VS range from 22% to 64.2%.[2,10] Given this high rate, the first treatment decision has often already been made based on the presumption of being a VS. As MRI resolution continues to improve, it is hoped this rate will decline.

Like VS, FNS are slow-growing lesions. Rates of growth have been reported to be between 0.85 and 1.4 mm per year.[3,8] As such, most authors recommend conservative management with serial imaging when symptoms are minimal and the FN function remains better than House-Brackmann (HB) grade III.[2,3,10,11] In several reports, FNSs have been followed for more than 5 years before requiring intervention.[2,3] Those patients who never required intervention have been able to maintain their baseline HB function with no impact on hearing.[2,3] This is the ideal patient outcome, but unfortunately not always possible because of tumor growth and worsening symptoms.

Angeli and Brackmann[9] introduced FNS decompression as a more conservative surgical treatment to preserve FN integrity and relieve pressure to allow improved axonal flow (**Fig. 4**). This seems to be an effective measure to allow FNS to continue to grow, but at a slow pace and with less neuronal injury. Multiple patients have been able to be treated with decompression without significant decreases in FN function over time.[3,11]

Wilkinson and colleagues[3] reported 19 patients treated with FN decompression with a mean 6-year follow-up. Four patients (21.0%) showed a decline in FN function by one HB grade over time and three showed improved HB grade.[3] There was also an increase in pure tone average by a mean 4.0 dB over this time period. These patients also showed decreased FNS growth rates of 0.17 mm per year compared with 0.85 mm per year in the observation cohort.[3] Similar results from the University of Iowa showed continued normal FN function 2 years after FNS decompression.[11] FN decompression has become a reasonable option in patients with growing bone-confined FNS and worsening FN function.

Although first introduced by Pulec in 1972,[13] FNS tumor debulking remains controversial. The histologic evidence of FN fibers running throughout FNS in tumor specimens has caused some to reject this treatment method.[14,15] Nevertheless there are

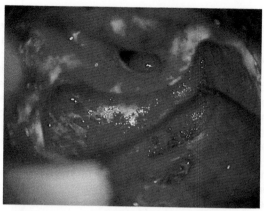

Fig. 4. Facial nerve schwannoma during transmastoid decompression procedure. Tumor involving tympanic segment and second genu of the facial nerve (instruments pointing to the lesion).

numerous reports in the literature showing good FN outcomes using debulking for FNS.[2,4,10,11,13,16,17] Supporters of debulking surgery believe that given advances in FN monitoring technology, portions of tumor that do not directly stimulate can be removed until fibrillation potentials are seen.[4,11] Unfortunately, FN stimulation at the end of the case has not been shown to be predictive of FN outcome in these cases.[2] Based on tumor size and location, patient symptomology, and preoperative hearing, FNS debulking can be performed either through a middle cranial fossa, transmastoid, translabyrinthine, or combined approach.

Mowry and colleagues[11] reported on 11 patients with FNS isolated to IAC and CPA that underwent debulking. They were able to perform 95% tumor removal in nine patients (81.8%), 80% removal in one (9.1%), and 66% tumor removal in one (9.1%). One patient who was lost to follow-up had a preoperative HB grade I but developed an HB grade IV in the immediate postoperative period. Otherwise, multiple patients who preoperatively had HB grade III or worse improved their FN function to an HB grade I to II after surgery. Only one patient (10%) developed an HB grade III with a mean follow-up of 28.2 months (range, 2–96 months). One patient did develop tumor recurrence that required complete resection of the FNS with an FN graft.[11]

In a recent study, Park and colleagues[10] attempted to identify factors to determine the best candidates for debulking surgery. Of the 28 patients undergoing surgery for FNS, 18 (64.3%) underwent FNS debulking. Of these 18 patients, two (11.1%) developed worse than HB grade III function. They identified several factors that they believed allowed them to perform tumor debulking with minimal postoperative FN injury. Patients with good outcomes, considered HB grade I to II after debulking, were more likely to have tumors less than 2 cm; two or less involved FN segments, and had tumors proximal to and including the GG. Because of the small sample size, however, none of these factors reach statistical significance. One patient (5.6%) had continued growth of residual tumor and required stereotactic radiation therapy.[10]

Data on subtotal tumor resection are sparse, but do show that a subset of patients can maintain good FN function postoperatively. Long-term follow-up is required to determine the viability of this option for FNS treatment. In the paper with the longest follow-up (mean, 7 years), Li and colleagues[4] reported they were able to perform

95% tumor resection in 10 patients and 70% to 80% resection in five patients. Overall, 27% of patient showed tumor growth over time. This rate increased to 60% when looking only at those undergoing 70% to 80% debulking. Although the sample size was small there was a clear trend toward increased likelihood of growth in those undergoing smaller percentage resections. This is helpful in counseling patients after surgery, but does not help in the treatment decision-making process because it is impossible to know the extent of safe tumor debulking before surgery.[4]

Patients presenting with poor FN function (>HB grade III) are less difficult treatment decisions. In this group with enlarging tumors, complete resection of the FNS with FN graft is the best option. For this population, outcome expectation should be lowered because the best possible outcome with an FN graft is HB grade III. In such cases, FN function has been shown to be improved or the same in 52% to 55% of patients, with 84% having HB grade III or IV.[2,3] Collagen nerve tubules have been used recently and may help improve FN outcomes in this population. Difficulty arises in these cases, however, when the FN is found to be involved at the brainstem, without a proximal stump, and is thus not amenable to grafting. In such cases, FN reanimation procedures are valuable.

Independent studies by the authors have shown a substantial change in the management of FNS over time.[2,3] Data from the House Ear Clinic show that before 1995, 85% of diagnosed FNS underwent resection, 15% decompression, and 0% observation. In contrast, in those diagnosed after 1995 only 27% underwent resection, 32.7% decompression, and 29% observation.[3] A similar pattern of more conservative management was also reported from the Otology Group of Vanderbilt. Here the number of FNS resections with graft decreased from 74% to 40% and the number of subtotal resections increased from 2.1% to 30% over a similar time period.[2] As the understanding of these tumors improves, the treatment algorithm is likely to continue to evolve.

A more recent addition to the management of FNS is the application of stereotactic radiosurgery (SRS). Unfortunately, like VS SRS literature, early reports on its effectiveness used vague terms for tumor control, hearing, balance, and FN outcomes. Recently, standard outcomes measures have been used with increased frequency. The full range of SRS techniques have been used to treat FNS with tumor control rates ranging from 83.3% to 100%.[2,3,18–24] In most patients, FN function has remained unchanged, but there are multiple reports of FN function worsening after treatment.[3,18,19,24]

One of the main factors that make understanding the outcomes of SRS for FNS difficult is that a large percentage of patients in the literature had surgery before their radiation therapy where the FNS was initially thought to be a VS. Presumptively, these patients then underwent decompression surgeries without tumor resection. We have previously discussed that FNSs undergoing decompression show slower rates of growth. Likewise, FN injury from post-SRS tumor swelling is presumably less likely if a decompression is performed. Therefore, separating the outcomes in those previously treated with surgery and not is difficult given the small patient population. Long-term data are needed to determine the efficacy of this treatment.

GENICULATE GANGLION HEMANGIOMAS

Hemangiomas involving the FN invariably arise from the GG leading many to term these lesions GGHs. These lesions represent just 0.7% of intratemporal vascular lesions.[25] Although termed hemangiomas throughout the literature, these lesions likely do not represent classic infantile hemangiomas. Rather, McKenna-Benoit and colleagues[26] showed that these lesions histologically showed irregular dilated vessels lacking internal elastic lamina with scant associated smooth muscle. In addition these lesions lacked GLUT1 and LewisY staining making hemangioma a less likely diagnosis.[26] Given the more common use of hemangioma in the literature, however, we use that term in this article.

GGHs arise from the extensive capillary plexus surrounding the GG.[27] These are slow-growing lesions that are noted to show FN paralysis out of proportion to their size. Progressive FN paralysis occurs in 90% of patients presenting with these lesions compared with 5% who present with sudden onset.[28] This can lead to delayed diagnosis if the cause is presumed to be Bell palsy. Facial twitch has also been noted to occur in a significant number of patients. As GGHs grow, they can cause a cochlear fistula leading to a sensorineural hearing loss; this can be seen in nearly 25% of patients.[25,28]

Imaging is key to diagnosing FN hemangiomas, with MRI being the most sensitive imaging technique.[29] On MRI, they show a heterogeneous hyperintensitiy on T2-weighted imaging with stippled punctate foci of hypointense signal confined, more frequently, to the GG. Rarely, these tumors can be present in the IAC, and seen as heterogeneous contrast-enhancing lesions on T1-weighted imaging with punctate areas of nonenhancement that correspond to ossified foci (**Fig. 5**). Given that 80% are less than 1 cm,[28] GGH can easily be overlooked. When high suspicion exists, a CT can be helpful in diagnosis. Unlike schwannomas, GGH have irregular borders and intratumoral bone spicules. This intratumoral bone formation is thought to arise from a reaction from the surrounding bone.[30]

Treatment of GGH has changed over time. The traditional method was to wait until the patient developed severe FN paralysis and perform resection of the involved portion of the FN with a cable graft repair. More recent data have supported a technique that removes the GGH while leaving the FN intact.[26,28] Semaan and colleagues[28] reported improved FN outcomes using this method over FN resection

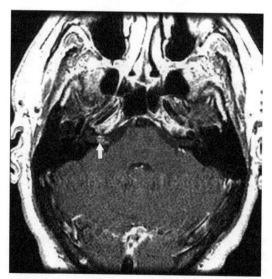

Fig. 5. Facial nerve hemangioma of the IAC. T1-weighted MRI with contrast, axial view, showing a right heterogeneous lesion with stippled punctate foci of hypointense signal that correspond to intratumoral bony spicules (*arrow*).

and grafting. In their series of 15 patients, 13 underwent middle fossa approach and two translabyrinthine because of lack of serviceable hearing. Eleven patients had anatomically preserved FN, all of whom had postoperative HB grade III or better. Of the four patients undergoing FN excision with grafting, only one achieved HB grade III. Hearing was unchanged in 64% of patients in this group. Interestingly, two patients had a fistula into to middle turn of the cochlear noted intraoperatively that was not seen on preoperative imaging.[28]

The diagnosis of GGH should be considered in any patient with FN paralysis out of proportion to their tumor size. Optimal treatment methods for GGH are hard to determine given the small number of reports in the literature. Based on the available data, these should be monitored if noted incidentally without FN paralysis or hearing loss. When FN paralysis is initially noted (HB grade III or worse) a middle cranial fossa FN-sparing resection should be performed if hearing is serviceable and through a translabyrinthine approach if not.

GLOMUS FACIALIS

Within the temporal bone, glomus tympanicum and glomus jugulare represent most paraganglioma. As these lesions grow, the FN can become secondarily involved. There are several cases in the literature, however, of glomus tumors arising primarily in the fallopian canal and directly invading the FN.[31–33] Most of these tumors have been identified in the vertical portion of the FN near the jugular bulb and stylomastoid foramen.[31,33]

In the few reported cases, FN paralysis seems to be the most common presenting symptom followed by pulsatile tinnitus.[31–33] Imaging characteristics on CT and MRI are similar to those of other paraganglioma with bony destruction, high T2 signal, and marked enhancement with "salt and pepper" appearance on T1 with gadolinium contrast. The sole method of isolating these lesions as glomus facialis is by the absence of involvement of the middle ear and jugular bulb. These tumors can be treated conservatively without resection until FN paralysis occurs. On histology, glomus facialis show the characteristic Zellballen pattern of other paraganglioma.[34]

GRANULAR CELL TUMORS

Like FNS, granular cell tumors arise from Schwann cells. Overall, most granular cell tumors are found in the tongue.[35] They have a higher disposition in the fourth and fifth decades of life and in African Americans and women.[36] Histologically these tumor cells contain eosinophillic granules that stain positive with periodic acid–Schiff stain.

There is no clear treatment algorithm for granular cell tumors of the FN. Some have recommended being more aggressive than FNS because of their tendency to grow and the low, but present, risk of malignant degeneration.[37] When removed, complete resection with margins is recommended because of a 5% to 15% risk of recurrence.[37]

SUMMARY

Primary tumors of the FN are rare but pose a difficult treatment challenge when encountered. Each tumor can typically be diagnosed based on imaging, but choosing the optimal treatment option is difficult because the literature is sparse and often inconsistent. It is clear, however, that treatment of FNS has become more conservative over time. As more data on primary tumors of the FN are published, the treatment algorithm will continue to evolve in hopes of optimal patient outcomes.

REFERENCES

1. Saito H, Baxter A. Undiagnosed intratemporal facial nerve neurilemomas. Arch Otolaryngol 1972;95:415–9.
2. McRackan TR, Rivas AR, Wanna GB, et al. Facial nerve outcomes in facial nerve schwannomas. Otol Neurotol 2011;33:78–82.
3. Wilkinson EP, Hoa M, Slattery WH, et al. Evolution in the management of facial nerve schwannoma. Laryngoscope 2011;121:2065–74.
4. Li Y, Liu H, Cheng Y. Subtotal resection of facial nerve schwannoma is not safe in the long run. Acta Otolaryngol 2014;134:433–6.
5. Alyono JC, Corrales CE, Gurgel RK, et al. Facial nerve schwannomas presenting as occluding external auditory canal masses: a therapeutic dilemma. Otol Neurotol 2014;35(7):1284–9.
6. McMonagle B, Al-Sanosi A, Croxson G, et al. Facial schwannoma: results of a large case series and review. J Laryngol Otol 2008;122:1139–50.
7. O'Donoghue G, Brackmann D, House J, et al. Neuromas of the facial nerve. Am J Otol 1989;10:49–54.
8. Perez R, Chen JM, Nedzelski JM. Intratemporal facial nerve schwannoma: a management dilemma. Otol Neurotol 2005;26:121–6.
9. Angeli SI, Brackmann DE. Is surgical excision of facial nerve schwannomas always indicated? Otolaryngol Head Neck Surg 1997;117:S144–7.
10. Park SH, Kim J, Moon IS, et al. The best candidates for nerve-sparing stripping surgery for facial nerve schwannoma. Laryngoscope 2014;124(11):2610–5.
11. Mowry S, Hansen M, Gantz B. Surgical management of internal auditory canal and cerebellopontine angle facial nerve schwannoma. Otol Neurotol 2012;33:1071–6.
12. Antoni NR. Uber ruckenmarkstumoren und neurofibrome. Studien zur pathologischen anatomie und embryogenese. Munich (Germany): Bergman; 1920.
13. Pulec JL. Facial nerve neuroma. Laryngoscope 1972;82:1160–76.
14. Hajjaj M, Linthicum FH Jr. Facial nerve schwannoma: nerve fibre dissemination. J Laryngol Otol 1996;110:632–3.
15. Jung TT, Jun BH, Shea D, et al. Primary and secondary tumors of the facial nerve. A temporal bone study. Arch Otolaryngol Head Neck Surg 1986;112:1269–73.
16. McMenomey SO, Glasscock ME, Minor LB, et al. Facial nerve neuromas presenting as acoustic tumors. Am J Otol 1994;15:307–12.
17. Sherman JD, Dagnew E, Pensak M, et al. Facial nerve neuromas: report of 10 cases and review of the literature. Neurosurgery 2002;50:450–6.
18. Kida Y, Yoshimoto M, Hasegawa T. Radiosurgery for facial schwannoma. J Neurosurg 2007;106:24–9.
19. Litre CF, Gourg GP, Tamura M, et al. Gamma knife surgery for facial nerve schwannomas. Neurosurgery 2007;60:853–9.
20. Hillman TA, Chen DA, Fuhrer R. An alternative treatment for facial nerve tumors: short-term results of radiotherapy. Ear Nose Throat J 2008;87:574–7.
21. Ingrosso A, Ponti E, di Cristino D, et al. Intra-parotid facial nerve schwannoma with intra-temporal extension; a case report. Is there a role for stereotactic radiotherapy? Am J Otolaryngol 2013;34:258–61.
22. Madhok R, Kondziolka D, Flickinger JC, et al. Gamma knife radiosurgery for facial schwannomas. Neurosurgery 2009;64:1102–5.
23. Nishioka K, Abo D, Aoyama H, et al. Stereotactic radiotherapy for intracranial nonacoustic schwannomas including facial nerve schwannoma. Int J Radiat Oncol Biol Phys 2009;75:1415–9.

24. Jacob JT, Driscoll CL, Link MJ. Facial nerve schwannomas of the cerebellopontine angle: the Mayo Clinic experience. J Neurol Surg B Skull Base 2012;73: 230–5.
25. Mangham CA, Carberry JN, Brackmann DE. Management of intratemporal vascular tumors. Laryngoscope 1981;91:867–76.
26. McKenna-Benoit M, North PE, McKenna MJ, et al. Facial nerve hemangiomas: vascular tumors or malformations? Otolaryngol Head Neck Surg 2010;142: 108–44.
27. El-Khouly H, Fernandez-Miranda J, Rhoton AL Jr. Blood supply of the facial nerve in the middle fossa: the petrosal artery. Neurosurgery 2008;62:297–303.
28. Semaan MT, Slattery WH, Brackmann DE. Geniculate ganglion hemangiomas: clinical results and long-term follow-up. Otol Neurotol 2010;31:665–70.
29. Lo WW, Shelton C, Waluch V, et al. Intratemporal vascular tumors: detection with CT and MR imaging. Radiology 1989;171:445–8.
30. Gavilan J, Nistal M, Gavilan C, et al. Ossifying hemangioma of the temporal bone. Arch Otolaryngol Head Neck Surg 1990;116:965–7.
31. Dutcher PO, Brackmann DE. Glomus tumor of the facial canal. Arch Otolaryngol Head Neck Surg 1986;112:986–7.
32. Petrus LV, Lo WM. Primary paraganglioma of the facial nerve canal. AJNR Am J Neuroradiol 1996;17(1):171–4.
33. Sanchez-Cuadrado I, Lassaletta L, Gonzalez-Otero T, et al. Radiology quiz case: glomus facialis paraganglioma. JAMA Otolaryngol Head Neck Surg 2013;139(1): 94–5.
34. Mafee MF, Raofi B, Kumar A, et al. Glomus faciale, glomus jugulare, glomus tympanicum, glomus vagale, carotid body tumors, and simulating lesions: role of MR imaging. Radiol Clin North Am 2000;38(5):1059–76.
35. Lack EE, Worsham GF, Callihan MD, et al. Granular cell tumor: a clinicopathologic study of 110 patients. J Surg Oncol 1980;13:301–16.
36. May M, Beckford NS, Bedetti CD. Granular cell tumor of facial nerve diagnosed at surgery for idiopathic facial nerve paralysis. Otolaryngol Head Neck Surg 1985; 93:122–6.
37. Lerut B, Vosbeck J, Linder TE. A forgotten facial nerve tumour: granular cell tumour of the parotid and its implications for treatment. J Laryngol Otol 2011; 125(4):410–4.

Chordoma and Chondrosarcoma

Jamie J. Van Gompel, MD[a],*, Jeffrey R. Janus, MD[b]

KEYWORDS

- Chondrosarcoma • Chordoma • Outcome • Proton beam • Surgery

KEY POINTS

- Chordomas are locally aggressive tumors derived from notochord remnants.
- Chondrosarcomas are generally low-grade, indolent malignancies that cause morbidity through compression of neurovascular structures at the skull base.
- The primary treatment of both chordoma and chondrosarcoma is aggressive primary resection followed by adjuvant radiation therapy.
- Heavy particle therapy, such as proton beam or carbon ion, provides higher treatment doses with less toxicity and currently is most commonly recommended for chordomas and chondrosarcomas after surgical resection.
- Chordomas and chondrosarcomas create multifaceted clinical challenges and should be managed by multidisciplinary skull base teams with expertise in their treatment.

Videos of chordoma and chondrosarcoma surgeries accompany this article at http://www.oto.theclinics.com/

INTRODUCTION

Chordoma and chondrosarcoma have been grouped together historically because of the midline presentation, similar radiography, and confusion in initial pathology. However, these lesions are distinct clinicopathological entities and vary significantly in their clinical outcome. Both lesions are uncommon and represent less than 1% of intracranial lesions.[1,2] Each poses a daunting challenge to effective treatment due to the perilous proximity of critical cranial nerves, the brainstem, and the skull base vasculature. To that end, both tumors have a tendency to recur locally, even after aggressive resection, especially if known residual tumor is left behind. Chordomas may metastasize

Disclosures: The authors report no conflicts of interests.
a Departments of Neurosurgery and Otolaryngology, Mayo Clinic, 200 First Street, Southwest, Rochester, MN 55905, USA; b Division of Otolaryngology Head and Neck Surgery, Department of Otolaryngology, Mayo Clinic, Rochester, MN 55905, USA
* Corresponding author.
E-mail address: vangompel.jamie@mayo.edu

Otolaryngol Clin N Am 48 (2015) 501–514
http://dx.doi.org/10.1016/j.otc.2015.02.009
0030-6665/15/$ – see front matter © 2015 Elsevier Inc. All rights reserved.

oto.theclinics.com

Abbreviations

Gy   Gray
WHO   World Health Organization

with time; however, they rarely present as such. Despite these concerns, the combination of maximal resection with minimal morbidity, followed by aggressive high-dose postoperative radiation therapy, can cure most low-grade chondrosarcomas, and provides good long-term local control and quality of life in patients with chordoma and high-grade chondrosarcoma.

Chordomas are malignant primary bone tumors that are derived from notochord remnants. They were first recognized in 1856 by Lushka and concomitantly by Virchow in 1857 at autopsy.[3,4] Originally thought to be of cartilaginous origin, Muller proposed these tumors were derived from notochord in 1958.[5] The term chordoma was later suggested after these tumors were directly observed in the nucleus pulposis, incriminating their origin.[6] They occur in the axial skeleton, where the notochord resides developmentally. Their occurrence in the axial spine can be thought of in terms of thirds, with a third arising in the skull base, spine, and sacrum 32%, 33%, and 29% of patients, respectively. It should be noted, however, that other studies support a more caudal cranial distribution of cases with less axial spine involvement.[7] Chordoma has an incidence of 8.4 cases per 10 million population in the United States.[7] They frequently recur locally despite aggressive surgical treatment. Although metastases do occur, these are uncommon and are not frequently existent at initial presentation. Ecchordosis physaliphora, which is also a remnant of the embryonic notochord, is a different entity and is found typically intradurally behind the clivus and anterior to the brainstem.[8,9] Pathologically, ecchordosis physaliphora is virtually identical to chordoma.[8,9] In the context of a patient, however, these are commonly smaller; there is complete lack of clival involvement, and they frequently follow a benign clinical course.[8,9]

Chondrosarcomas are rare cartilaginous tumors that may present as low grade (World Health Organization [WHO] 1 or 2), which are far and away more common, or high grade (WHO grade 3), as well as a mesenchymal chordoma subtype. WHO grade 3 and mesenchymal subtype tumors forbear a worse prognosis.[1,2] Only 1% of chondrosarcomas occur at the skull base.[10] The cell of origin is unknown; however, typically these are thought to arise from synchodroses of the skull base, such as the spheno-occipital suture or petroclival suture. They frequently present eccentric, but do not stray far from midline.[1,2] Sixty-six percent of skull base chondrosarcomas arise from the petroclival fissure; an additional 28% percent arise from the clivus proper, and a further 6% arise from the sphenoethmoidal complex.[11] The lattermost of these is a fusion plane, which is off midline, accounting for eccentric presentation just lateral to midline. Chondrosarcomas are typically less aggressive than chordomas, rarer, and very uncommonly metastasize.[1,2]

PRESENTING CHARACTERISTICS
Chordoma

These are the most common extradural clival tumors. The median age of presentation for skull base chordomas appears to be 60 years of age; however, there is a large range of presenting ages, including pediatric cases.[7,12–15] Chordomas produce morbidity and mortality through local growth. Often upper clival chordomas will present with sixth nerve palsies secondary to the tumor accessing the basilar venous plexus between the periosteal and parietal dural layers producing a local compartment syndrome of dorello's canal. However, other cranial neuropathies can be seen with cavernous sinus involvement, including third and less commonly fourth nerve palsies. Headache is another frequent presenting symptom, and in larger tumors, nasal obstruction can be seen as well as eustachian tube dysfunction. If there is brainstem compression, there may be imbalance or hemiparesis as a presenting symptom. Lower clival tumors can present with dysphagia due to mass effect or involvement of the lower cranial nerves. There is no association known between chordomas and environmental exposures or radiation induction of chordomas.[1,2] There are no associated syndromes of which chordomas are a part; however, the investigation of (T) bracyury, brachyury duplication, and tuberous sclerosis complex are being investigated with respect to genetic predisposition.[1,2,16–18]

Chondrosarcoma

Chondrosarcoma is less common than chordoma, particularly in the setting of skull base tumors. In combined series, the occurrence is typically one-half to one-third the frequency of chordomas. Interpretation of incidence is a bit confounding due to the fact that older combined series may have mistaken chondrosarcoma for chondroid chordomas, while now this distinction is more clear.[1,2] The presenting characteristics for chondrosarcoma are similar to those stated previously for chordomas. Eccentric location, however, gives a slightly higher rate of cavernous sinus involvement, and associated diplopias are more frequent. Although chondrosarcomas typically occur in isolation, unlike chordomas, they can be associated with Paget disease, Ollier disease, and Maffuci syndrome.[11,19]

IMAGING
Chordomas

Imaging characteristics are fairly uniform for chordomas (**Fig. 1**). Classically they appear hyperintense on T2 weighted MRI.[20] On T1 weighted MRI, they are somewhat heterogeneous, with a predominantly hypointense signal.[21] Gadolinium enhancement is variable. The authors' own historical institutional data of over 30 skull base chordomas demonstrate minimal enhancement in 45% of cases, normal enhancement in 30% of cases, and avid enhancement in 25% of cases. Diffusion restriction is seen; however, the bony interfaces of the skull base make this finding unreliable. Thirty percent of cases demonstrate calcifications within the tumor. Dural transgression occurs 50% of the time at presentation. In terms of anatomic localization, 80% of cases demonstrate posterior clinoid involvement; 30% have occipital condylar involvement. Seventy percent of cases have cavernous sinus involvement; involvement of the upper half of the clivus occurs in 95% of cases, and the lower half of the clivus is involved in 30% of cases.

Chondrosarcomas

Imaging characteristics are similar to chordomas in that bright signal on T2 is a hallmark characteristic (**Fig. 2**).[20] As stated previously, chondrosarcomas are more eccentric to midline but are by no means lateral skull base lesions. Chondrosarcomas have variable World Health Organization (WHO) grades from 1 to 3; however, there does not appear to be any imaging hallmarks to differentiate low-grade from high-grade chondrosarcomas.

PATHOLOGY

Grossly, chordomas are lobulated and greyish-to-dark tumors. They can be firm with calcifications; however, in one author's (Van Gompel) they experience, typically are

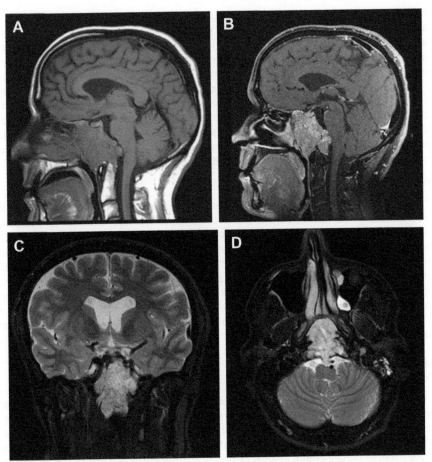

Fig. 1. Classic appearing clival chordoma occupying the entire clivus with minor dural transgression. (*A*) Sagittal T1-weighted MRI. (*B*) Sagital T1 with gadolinium. (*C*) Coronal and (*D*) axial T2 images demonstrating the classic-appearing T2 hyperintensity.

gelatinous and suckable. Chordoma can come in one of 3 histologic subtypes, namely classical (conventional), chondroid, and dedifferentiated.[1,2] They stain positive for brachyury, which links it to its cell of origin, the notochord. These tumors stain positive for S-100 and epithelial membrane antigen (EMA).[1,2] Virchow himself first described this tumor with intracellular bubble-like inclusions, also known as physaliferous cells, which are essentially pathognomonic for this tumor.[4] Unlike chondroid chordoma, chondrosarcomas are nonreactive for keratin and epithelial membrane antigen.[1,2] Chondrosarcomas may have a gross appearance much like chordomas, but more frequently are firm, and calcifications occur within them. Histologically low-grade tumors again are difficult to distinguish from chordoma, while higher grade tumors are not, and a variant, the mesenchymal subtype, is considered a more aggressive chondrosarcoma.[2] The grading is based on the degree of cellularity, atypia, and mitotic activity. In a large series of 200 patients, 51% were grade 1; 21% were grade 2, and 29% were a mixed grade 1 and 2. There were no grade 3 tumors seen.[11]

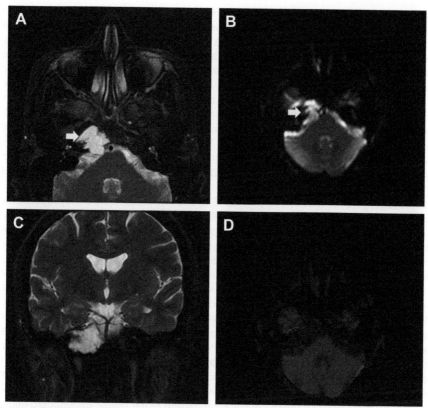

Fig. 2. Chondrosarcoma (*arrows* in *A, B*) residing in the right petrous apex and petroclival fissure: T2-weighted axial (*A*) and coronal (*C*) MRI demonstrating a smaller petrous apex chondrosarcoma with high T2 signal intensity. Diffusion weighted imaging (DWI) (*B*) demonstrates the lesion to be diffusion restricting, which may confuse it with epidermoid or petrous apex cholesteatoma. When viewing DWI, it is important to ensure that there is no T2 shine through on the apparent diffusion coefficient (ADC) map as shown here (*D*). This lesion underwent an endonasal approach with a 90% resection, leaving a small residual on the backside of the carotid and proved to be a chondrosarcoma.

MANAGEMENT
Surgery

Chordomas and chondrosarcomas

Both chordomas and chondrosarcomas should be treated by a multidisciplinary skull base team including neurosurgery, otolaryngology, medical oncology, and radiation oncology, with participation also coming from endocrinology, ophthalmology, and rehabilitation (Videos 1 and 2). Although en bloc resection is frequently the goal in the sacrum and the spine, rarely can a chordoma of the skull base be taken out in such a manner. Philosophy regarding the removal of these tumors has greatly evolved in recent decades, with resection in a piecemeal fashion considered to be oncologically sound. Frequently, in older series, simple biopsy was performed with intralesional curettage. The recent advent of skull base techniques and even more recent cultivation of endoscopic techniques have permitted more thorough removal of tumor with less postoperative morbidity. Certain authors have taken this to the extreme and advocate resection of as much of the clivus as possible during primary surgery with potential staged operations to achieve this, citing the frequency of recurrence as the primary reason.[22–24] The current authors' stance is similar in that all boney involvement and adjacent bone that can be safely taken should be; however, cavernous sinus involvement often precludes complete resection, and few authors have advocated carotid resection because of high morbidity. In turn, adjuvant radiation can be used to treat residual tumor. It should be noted that aggressive surgical series document a higher rate of carotid injury, which may indicate that chordomas themselves locally invade the carotid artery, potentially leading to higher carotid artery injuries in the operating room. This also may be related to the aggressive attempts at resection.[25–27] The authors advocate a plan to deal with intraoperative carotid bleeding, and in select cases perform preoperative balloon occlusion studies in preparation for such a catastrophic vascular injury.[26]

Lesions of the lower clivus pose a similar dilemma in that complete boney resection in this area may impart occipital cervical instability. In younger and healthier patients, however, complete resection with concomitant posterior fusion may be an option to obtain better margin status.[28] Typically, if the dura is not invaded, it is left in situ as a barrier; however, if there is dural transgression, the authors advocate dural resection with a negative margin goal. Brainstem involvement is managed with resection of the capsule of the tumor, but brainstem margins are not taken. In cases of cranial nerve involvement, hypoglossal being the most frequent conundrum, resection of this nerve is only undertaken if there is an opportunity for complete resection. The authors do not advocate bilateral hypoglossal sacrifice if there is bilateral involvement due to the morbidity of such a resection to the patient. The sixth nerve is also frequently involved in Dorello canal; however, in such circumstances, the authors typically perform decompression, resecting the tumor around the nerve but not the nerve itself. Although the approach to each tumor is variable depending on size and location, an anterior approach is favored, because most of these tumors arise midline in the clivus. Endoscopic endonasal approaches generally allow access from the frontal recess to the base of C2. Advanced endoscopic approaches, such as the transpterygoid procedure, the extradural pituitary transposition (**Fig. 3**), the petrous apex approach (**Fig. 4**), and the far medial approach (**Fig. 5**) can be employed to achieve complete resection of tumor.[29–31]

The most challenging hurdle encountered with endoscopic approaches to these tumors is defect closure and prevention of cerebrospinal fluid (CSF) leak. This has been aided substantially with the use of the nasoseptal flap. Even more formidable is the challenge in cases in which the nasoseptal flap cannot be harvested because of previous operation or tumor contamination. Such cases may require a more classical multilayer closure (see **Fig. 4**). In some circumstances, traditional transfacial approaches may be used to access difficult skull base chordomas. These situations are dwindling, however, in the shadow of more aggressive endoscopic endeavors. The role for transoral approaches is reserved for cases in which there is a low riding odontoid relative to the hard palate. Transoral approaches do have a higher association with postoperative dysphagia, however, when compared with endonasal approaches.[32,33] Certainly, disease lateral to the carotid will require traditional lateral skull base approaches such as anterior or posterior petrosectomy as well as other transtemporal variants, therefore, again emphasizing the role of multidisciplinary teams.

Lower clival tumors can also be reached by far or extreme lateral approaches. Other open approaches remain necessary to address tumors lateral to the carotid arteries. Chondrosarcomas appear to be more indolent than chordomas, which may lend to favoring a more conservative initial surgery. To that end, some small tumors and other select cases may be addressed with observation. Furthermore, in select cases of

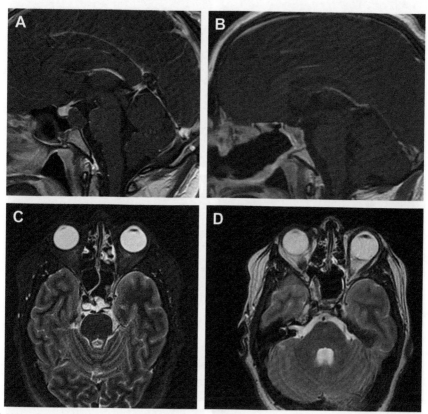

Fig. 3. Preoperative (*A, C*) and postoperative (*B, D*) images of a chordoma, completely removed endoscopically with an interdural pituitary transposition and repair with nasoseptal flap.

chondrosarcoma in which there is little to no preoperative growth, residual tumor can be observed closely without adjuvant treatment; this is because local recurrence rates and ability to metastasize are less than chordoma. In the end, with either chordoma or chondrosarcoma, the surgical and adjuvant treatment plan should be tailored to each patient to optimize outcome, with strong consideration of comorbidity and age.

Radiation Therapy

The role of adjuvant radiation is a matter of debate and is generally recommended after initial aggressive resection, especially with residual tumor. The type of radiation that should be used is also controversial. Conventional radiotherapy with doses between 50 and 60 Gray (Gy) demonstrate poor local control rates, ranging between 17% and 23% after 5 years.[34,35] Stereotactic fractionated radiation therapy appears to improve outcomes. With a median dose of 67 Gy, 5-year local control rates near 50% have been reported.[36] Currently, heavy particle and charged particle therapy are the most commonly recommended radiation treatments for chordoma and chondrosarcoma. Proton and carbon ion particle radiation have a theoretic advantage of sharp Bragg peak drop off at the tumor edge, which minimizes the radiation dose to the adjacent brainstem and allows higher treatment dose. However, this modality is frequently much more expensive than conventional radiation therapy, and it has poor availability

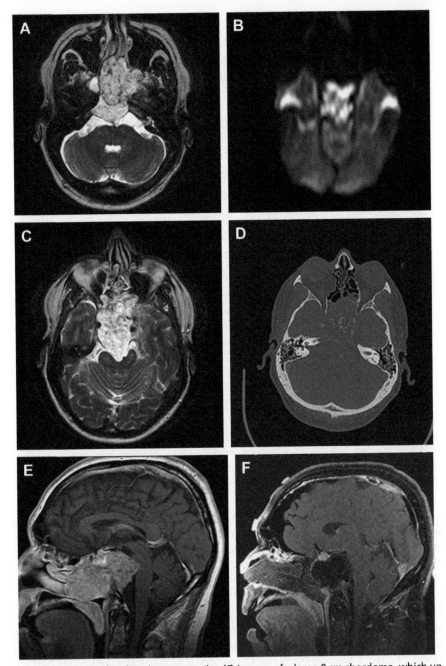

Fig. 4. Preoperative (*A–E*) and postoperative (*F*) images of a large 8 cm chordoma, which underwent complete resection with classic multilayer closure. Classic closure was performed due to tumor contamination of nasoseptal flaps. Preoperative T2 axial images (*A, C*) demonstrating classic high signal on T2 with dural transgression, midbrain compression, and invasion of the cavernous sinus as well as the pterygopalatine space. Diffusion weighted axial imaging (*B*) demonstrating diffusion restriction, a variable finding in chordomas. Axial computed tomography (CT) (*D*) showing intratumoral calcifications, which can be found in chordomas but are not typical. Sagittal preoperative T1 with gadolinium showing the contamination of the nasoseptal flaps and significant brainstem compression. Postoperative T1 with gadolinium and fat suppression showing the skull base reconstruction and complete resection.

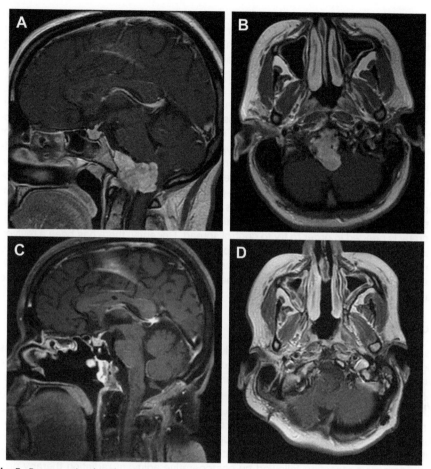

Fig. 5. Preoperative (*A, B*) and postoperative (*C, D*) MRI T1 sequence with gadolinium in the sagittal (*A, C*) and axial (*B, D*) of a formidable lower clivus chordoma requiring a endoscopic far medial as a stage one approach followed by a far lateral to achieve a gross total resection. The patient had no postoperative deficits.

to patients, who frequently have to travel great distances to receive this therapy at the limited number of current centers. Regardless, proton beam treatment in its present form appears to have a survival advantage, with the 5-year local control rate of 73% after 72 Gy. It should be noted that the aforementioned series may project an elevated level of local control due to a highly selected cohort with very little residual tumor upon treatment.[37] Carbon ion therapy is now available in Europe, and in addition to sharper radiation dropoff, heavy particle therapy may offer an additional advantage of biologic activity against tumors not traditionally responsive to photon-based radiation therapy.[38–41] Early results with carbon ion therapy reveal, when used adjuvantly to treat patients with residual tumor, a local control rate of 70% at 5 years.[38–41] There appears to be similar toxicities between the modalities if the dose limitations are kept in mind. Intensity-modulated radiation therapy is frequently used in areas where particle therapy is not available as the most current conventional radiation therapy and may offer a similar benefit; however, this has not been thoroughly investigated. Most current series studying long-term outcome with conventional radiation therapy employed older techniques and may not apply to current management. Finally, stereotactic radiosurgery using Gamma Knife, Cyberknife, or other similar units certainly plays a role in primary radiation therapy, particularly in smaller tumors. Stereotactic radiosurgery can also be employed in cases of residual or recurrent disease.

Chemotherapy

There are few available data demonstrating efficacy of any chemotherapeutic regimen in controlling these tumors, and much less showing any evidence of tumor size reduction. Therefore, most chemotherapeutic regimens are currently used in palliative or heroic efforts once surgical local control options are exhausted. These may be considered experimental on a patient-by-patient basis. There are no data available at the time of this publication demonstrating preoperative neoadjuvant therapy as a prelude to improving surgical margins. Due to the gravity of a surgically and radiation-resistant tumor, typically, chemotherapy regimens are similar to those used as sarcoma regimens and have shown little efficacy. Further, in cases of metastatic disease, chemotherapy is needed in order to try to control spread. Recently, there has been a revived enthusiasm in exploring molecular therapy for chordoma, as these tumors appear to have tyrosine kinase and related pathway mutations.[42] Chondrosarcomas rarely metastasize, and it is infrequent that one seeks adjuvant chemotherapy with these patients.

OUTCOME

As stated previously, historically the inclusion of chordomas and chondrosarcomas together is based on similar locations and overlap in pathology; however, in no place can more drastic differences be seen than in outcomes between these 2 pathologies.

Chordoma

If not treated, the natural history of chordoma is local progression, with an average survival of around 18 months.[43,44] Although there is significant variance in outcomes with isolated surgical resection or radiation therapy alone, it is generally accepted that aggressive resection followed by postoperative adjuvant radiation therapy provides the best long term outcomes. The median overall survival according to the most recent Surveillance, Epidemiology, and End Results Program (SEER) results is 7.7 years.[7] Patients presenting under the age of 40 appear to have a better long-term survival (68%) at 10 years compared with those older than 40 (43%).[7] According to these data, elderly patients have a more aggressive form of disease.[7] Several reports have demonstrated extent of resection improves long-term outcome. For near-total or total resections, 5-year overall survival is 6 times more likely compared with subtotal resections (93% compared with 15%).[45] There is evidence to suggest that the quality of life of postsurgical patients is less than the general population.[46]

Chondrosarcoma

With chondrosarcoma, there is a clear survival advantage in patients who undergo resection compared with observation.[13] However, again, there may be select patients in whom observation is chosen. Other important favorable factors in survival include female sex, smaller tumor size at presentation, and younger age at treatment, each being proven in multivariate models in large series.[13] WHO grade 3 and mesenchymal subtype pathology also portends a poorer prognosis.[2] Five-year mortality and 10-year mortality in the SEER database are reported at 87% and 68% respectively, although when considering only low-grade chondrosarcomas this is considerably higher.[13]

TUMOR RECURRENCE AND SALVAGE THERAPY

When chondrosarcoma and chordoma demonstrate progression after initial treatment, they often exhibit a slow but relentless local growth. Frequently revision resection can be performed with the goal of decompression for new deficits. Additionally, Gamma Knife treatment may be employed for local recurrences less than 3 cm in size.[47] Repeat palliative radiation may also be used and can halt progression temporarily. This is typically short lived, however, and there is an increased incidence of radiation-induced complications. Although isolated in use, there are case reports of local ablation using either laser or cryotherapy. This may aid in palliative treatment; however, this has yet to be employed in the skull base.[48]

SUMMARY

Chordomas and chondrosarcomas are both locally aggressive tumors with many similarities in presentation, radiography, and pathology. Although such similarities exist, differences in etiology, pathology, and prognosis abound, and these differences should be deeply considered in the management of each disease. In select circumstances, observation may be undertaken; however, primary surgical resection is considered the current standard of care. Radiation therapy is often recommended regardless of resection status. This recommendation is even stronger, however, in cases of tumor residual. Heavy ion radiation therapy is commonly suggested for postoperative adjuvant therapy; however, more data are needed before this becomes the standard of care. There are few options beyond repeat resection or stereotactic radiation for salvage therapy, as chemotherapy is uncommonly used for these tumors; however, future targeted therapies may hold promise as an additional treatment tool.

SUPPLEMENTARY DATA

Supplementary data related to this article can be found online at 10.1016/j.otc.2015.02.009.

REFERENCES

1. Central nervous system. 4th Edition. Lyon (France): International Agency for Research on Cancer: WHO Press; 2007.
2. Pathology and genetics of head and neck tumors. Lyon (France): International Agency for Research on Cancer: WHO Press; 2005.
3. Luschka H. Die Altersveranderungen der Zwischenwirbelknorpel. Virchows Arch Path Anat 1856;9:312–27.
4. Virchow R. Untersuchungen über die Entwickelung des Schadelgrundes im gesunden und krankhafter Zustande, und über den Einfluss derselben auf Schadelform, Gesichtsbildung und Gehirnbau. Berlin: G. Zeimer; 1857.
5. Muller H. Über das Vorkommen von Resten der Chorda dorsalis bei Mecschen nach der Geburt und uber ihr Verhaltnis zu den Gallertgeschwulsten am Clivus. Ztschr Rat Med 1858;2:202–29.
6. Ribbert H. Über die Ecchondrosis physlifora sphenooccipitalis. Centralbl Allg Path Path Anat 1894;5:457–61.
7. Smoll NR, Gautschi OP, Radovanovic I, et al. Incidence and relative survival of chordomas: the standardized mortality ratio and the impact of chordomas on a population. Cancer 2013;119:2029–37.

8. Ciarpaglini R, Pasquini E, Mazzatenta D, et al. Intradural clival chordoma and ecchordosis physaliphora: a challenging differential diagnosis: case report. Neurosurgery 2009;64:E387–8 [discussion: E388].

9. Iorgulescu JB, Laufer I, Hameed M, et al. Benign notochordal cell tumors of the spine: natural history of 8 patients with histologically confirmed lesions. Neurosurgery 2013;73:411–6.

10. Bloch O, Parsa AT. Skull base chondrosarcoma: evidence-based treatment paradigms. Neurosurg Clin N Am 2013;24:89–96.

11. Rosenberg AE, Nielsen GP, Keel SB, et al. Chondrosarcoma of the base of the skull: a clinicopathologic study of 200 cases with emphasis on its distinction from chordoma. Am J Surg Pathol 1999;23:1370–8.

12. Erdem E, Angtuaco EC, Van Hemert R, et al. Comprehensive review of intracranial chordoma. Radiographics 2003;23:995–1009.

13. Jones PS, Aghi MK, Muzikansky A, et al. Outcomes and patterns of care in adult skull base chordomas from the surveillance, epidemiology, and end results (SEER) database. J Clin Neurosci 2014;21:1490–6.

14. Menezes AH. Clival and craniovertebral junction chordomas. World Neurosurg 2014;81:690–2.

15. Tan NC, Naidoo Y, Oue S, et al. Endoscopic surgery of skull base chordomas. J Neurol Surg B Skull Base 2012;73:379–86.

16. Kelley MJ, Shi J, Ballew B, et al. Characterization of T gene sequence variants and germline duplications in familial and sporadic chordoma. Hum Genet 2014;133:1289–97.

17. Pillay N, Plagnol V, Tarpey PS, et al. A common single-nucleotide variant in T is strongly associated with chordoma. Nat Genet 2012;44:1185–7.

18. Yang XR, Ng D, Alcorta DA, et al. T (brachyury) gene duplication confers major susceptibility to familial chordoma. Nat Genet 2009;41:1176–8.

19. Boorstein JM, Spizarny DL. Case report 476: chondrosarcoma of base of skull (CBS). Skeletal Radiol 1988;17:208–11.

20. Bag AK, Chapman PR. Neuroimaging: intrinsic lesions of the central skull base region. Semin Ultrasound CT MR 2013;34:412–35.

21. Doucet V, Peretti-Viton P, Figarella-Branger D, et al. MRI of intracranial chordomas. Extent of tumour and contrast enhancement: criteria for differential diagnosis. Neuroradiology 1997;39:571–6.

22. Al-Mefty O, Kadri PA, Hasan DM, et al. Anterior clivectomy: surgical technique and clinical applications. J Neurosurg 2008;109:783–93.

23. Almefty K, Pravdenkova S, Colli BO, et al. Chordoma and chondrosarcoma: similar, but quite different, skull base tumors. Cancer 2007;110:2457–67.

24. Colli BO, Al-Mefty O. Chordomas of the skull base: follow-up review and prognostic factors. Neurosurg Focus 2001;10:E1.

25. Fernandez-Miranda JC, Gardner PA, Snyderman CH, et al. Clival chordomas: a pathological, surgical, and radiotherapeutic review. Head Neck 2014;36:892–906.

26. Gardner PA, Tormenti MJ, Pant H, et al. Carotid artery injury during endoscopic endonasal skull base surgery: incidence and outcomes. Neurosurgery 2013;73:261–9 [discussion: 269–70].

27. Koutourousiou M, Gardner PA, Tormenti MJ, et al. Endoscopic endonasal approach for resection of cranial base chordomas: outcomes and learning curve. Neurosurgery 2012;71:614–24 [discussion: 624–5].

28. Colli B, Al-Mefty O. Chordomas of the craniocervical junction: follow-up review and prognostic factors. J Neurosurg 2001;95:933–43.

29. Fernandez-Miranda JC, Gardner PA, Rastelli MM Jr, et al. Endoscopic endonasal transcavernous posterior clinoidectomy with interdural pituitary transposition. J Neurosurg 2014;121:91–9.

30. Fernandez-Miranda JC, Morera VA, Snyderman CH, et al. Endoscopic endonasal transclival approach to the jugular tubercle. Neurosurgery 2012;71:146–58 [discussion: 158–9].

31. Van Gompel JJ, Alikhani P, Tabor MH, et al. Anterior inferior petrosectomy: defining the role of endonasal endoscopic techniques for petrous apex approaches. J Neurosurg 2014;120:1321–5.

32. Van Abel KM, Mallory GW, Kasperbauer JL, et al. Transnasal odontoid resection: is there an anatomic explanation for differing swallowing outcomes? Neurosurg Focus 2014;37:E16.

33. Van Gompel JJ, Morris JM, Kasperbauer JL, et al. Cystic deterioration of the C1-2 articulation: clinical implications and treatment outcomes. J Neurosurg Spine 2011;14:437–43.

34. Catton C, O'Sullivan B, Bell R, et al. Chordoma: long-term follow-up after radical photon irradiation. Radiother Oncol 1996;41:67–72.

35. Romero J, Cardenes H, la Torre A, et al. Chordoma: results of radiation therapy in eighteen patients. Radiother Oncol 1993;29:27–32.

36. Debus J, Schulz-Ertner D, Schad L, et al. Stereotactic fractionated radiotherapy for chordomas and chondrosarcomas of the skull base. Int J Radiat Oncol Biol Phys 2000;47:591–6.

37. Munzenrider JE, Liebsch NJ. Proton therapy for tumors of the skull base. Strahlenther Onkol 1999;175(Suppl 2):57–63.

38. Schulz-Ertner D, Haberer T, Jakel O, et al. Radiotherapy for chordomas and low-grade chondrosarcomas of the skull base with carbon ions. Int J Radiat Oncol Biol Phys 2002;53:36–42.

39. Schulz-Ertner D, Karger CP, Feuerhake A, et al. Effectiveness of carbon ion radiotherapy in the treatment of skull-base chordomas. Int J Radiat Oncol Biol Phys 2007;68:449–57.

40. Schulz-Ertner D, Nikoghosyan A, Didinger B, et al. Carbon ion radiation therapy for chordomas and low grade chondrosarcomas—current status of the clinical trials at GSI. Radiother Oncol 2004;73(Suppl 2):S53–6.

41. Schulz-Ertner D, Nikoghosyan A, Thilmann C, et al. Carbon ion radiotherapy for chordomas and low-grade chondrosarcomas of the skull base. Results in 67 patients. Strahlenther Onkol 2003;179:598–605.

42. Akhavan-Sigari R, Gaab MR, Rohde V, et al. Expression of vascular endothelial growth factor receptor 2 (VEGFR-2), inducible nitric oxide synthase (iNOS), and Ki-M1P in skull base chordoma: a series of 145 tumors. Neurosurg Rev 2014;37:79–88.

43. Eriksson B, Gunterberg B, Kindblom LG. Chordoma. A clinicopathologic and prognostic study of a Swedish national series. Acta Orthop Scand 1981;52:49–58.

44. Heffelfinger MJ, Dahlin DC, MacCarty CS, et al. Chordomas and cartilaginous tumors at the skull base. Cancer 1973;32:410–20.

45. Ouyang T, Zhang N, Zhang Y, et al. Clinical characteristics, immunohistochemistry, and outcomes of 77 patients with skull base chordomas. World Neurosurg 2014;81:790–7.

46. Diaz RJ, Maggacis N, Zhang S, et al. Determinants of quality of life in patients with skull base chordoma. J Neurosurg 2014;120:528–37.

47. Kano H, Iyer A, Lunsford LD. Skull base chondrosarcoma radiosurgery: a literature review. Neurosurgery 2014;61(Suppl 1):155–8.

48. Kurup AN, Woodrum DA, Morris JM, et al. Cryoablation of recurrent sacrococcygeal tumors. J Vasc Interv Radiol 2012;23:1070–5.

Stereotactic Radiosurgery in the Management of Vestibular Schwannoma and Glomus Jugulare

Indications, Techniques, and Results

Jeffrey T. Jacob, MD[a], Bruce E. Pollock, MD[a,b],
Matthew L. Carlson, MD[c], Colin L.W. Driscoll, MD[a,c],
Michael J. Link, MD[a,c],*

KEYWORDS

- Stereotactic radiosurgery • Vestibular schwannoma • Glomus jugulare
- Skull base tumors

KEY POINTS

- Gamma knife radiosurgery provides excellent functional preservation and tumor control in long-term follow-up for select patients with vestibular schwannomas or glomus jugulare tumors.
- Excellent pretreatment hearing is the most reliable predictor of long-term hearing preservation following stereotactic radiosurgery.
- Long-term follow-up is necessary to critically assess outcome after stereotactic radiosurgery.

INTRODUCTION AND TECHNIQUE

Gamma Knife stereotactic radiosurgery (GKS) was first instituted at the Mayo Clinic in 1990, being the third Gamma Knife unit to be installed in the United States, resulting in extensive experience in treating lateral skull base tumors over the past 24 years.[1] The Leksell Gamma Knife (Elekta Instruments, Norcoss, GA) uses either 201 (models U, B, C, 4-C) or 192 (model Perfexion) fixed cobalt 60 radiation sources that can be collimated to radiation beams of 4-mm, 8-mm, 14-mm, or 18-mm ovoids with the earlier models.

[a] Department of Neurologic Surgery, Mayo Clinic School of Medicine, Mayo Clinic, 200 First Street Southwest, Rochester, MN 55905, USA; [b] Department of Radiation Oncology, Mayo Clinic School of Medicine, 200 First Street Southwest, Rochester, MN 55905, USA; [c] Department of Otolaryngology-Head and Neck Surgery, Mayo Clinic School of Medicine, 200 First Street Southwest, Rochester, MN 55905, USA
* Corresponding author. Department of Neurologic Surgery, Mayo Clinic, 200 First Street Southwest, Rochester, MN 55905, USA.
E-mail address: link.michael@mayo.edu

Otolaryngol Clin N Am 48 (2015) 515–526
http://dx.doi.org/10.1016/j.otc.2015.02.010
0030-6665/15/$ – see front matter © 2015 Elsevier Inc. All rights reserved.
oto.theclinics.com

The current Perfexion model allows the radiation to be collimated to 4-mm, 8-mm, or 16-mm ovoids of radiation and in addition each shot is divided into 8 sections of 24 beams of radiation that can potentially be completely blocked or collimated to the 4-mm, 8-mm, or 16-mm sizes to allow more complex shapes than just the original ovoids. This ability also has the advantage of allowing blocking patterns to potentially protect critical radiation-sensitive structures such as the cochlea or optic nerves and chiasm.

A 4-point stereotactic head frame is applied after infiltration of the pin sites with local anesthetic. Detailed stereotactic imaging of the tumor and adjacent critical temporal bone structures is then performed using MRI and computed tomography (CT). A post-gadolinium axial spoiled gradient recalled (SPGR) acquisition in the steady state MRI with 1-mm thick, volumetrically acquired slices (28–60 images) is performed to encompass the tumor and surrounding pertinent anatomy. The patient is then taken to the CT scanner where a noncontrast axial CT scan of the temporal bones is obtained with 1-mm thick slices. This technique allows the user to contour the bony cochlea and determine an accurate volumetric dose to the cochlea. In addition, this enables clinicians to minimize the image distortion of stereotactic MRI.[2,3] It also allows better delineation of tumor involvement into the temporal bone in patients with, for example, paragangliomas. This imaging is directly transferred to a computer workstation. MRI and CT can also be fused using the Gamma Plan software (Elekta Instruments, Norcross, GA). A conformal radiation dose plan is then developed using a combination of isocenters that are derived by way of collimators of various sizes and differential weighting, after which the treatment is performed (**Fig. 1**). Patients are dismissed following the procedure from the outpatient observation ward without restrictions. We obtain follow-up audiograms and MRI scans at 6-month intervals for the first year, then yearly for the next several years, eventually moving to MRI scans every 3 to 4 years if no evidence of tumor growth is detected.

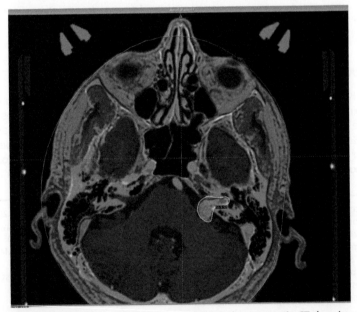

Fig. 1. Axial fused gadolinium-enhanced SPGR MRI and stereotactic CT showing the dose plan for a left-sided vestibular schwannoma (VS). The tumor margin dose was 12.5 Gy (*yellow outline*). Note the relationship of the cochlea (*purple outline*) to the 50% isodose line.

VESTIBULAR SCHWANNOMA TREATMENT
Dose

Dose planning and treatment of vestibular schwannoma (VS) have evolved significantly over the last several years, accounting for improved cranial nerve morbidity without compromising tumor control. During the early years of VS treatment at the Mayo Clinic, the mean tumor margin dose was 18 Gy (range, 16–20 Gy). Although tumor control was excellent, the rate of new facial weakness and the incidence of trigeminal neuropathy were high. Among 44 VSs treated between 1990 and 1993 the incidence of new facial weakness and facial paresthesias was 21% and 36% respectively. Moreover, the rate of serviceable hearing preservation during this time period was only 25%. In an effort to reduce cranial nerve morbidity, the prescribed tumor margin dose was reduced in 1994 and then again in 1996. At present, we typically prescribe 12 to 13 Gy for patients with serviceable hearing and 13 to 14 Gy for patients with poor pretreatment hearing. We treat using the 50% isodose line, which maintains a high intratumoral dose with steep radiation falloff.

Nonaudiologic Cranial Nerve Morbidity and Tumor Control

Between 1997 and 2000, 84 patients were treated with a mean tumor margin dose of 13 Gy at Mayo Clinic. Over this interval, there were no new cases of facial weakness, trigeminal symptoms occurred in less than 4% of patients, and the short-term serviceable hearing preservation rate improved to 77% compared with earlier treatment protocols.[4] In a prospective observational outcome analysis of 46 patients at our institution, comparing microsurgery with GKS for sporadic VS,[5] we saw facial weakness in 2 patients (4%) and 1 patient (2%) developed a new trigeminal neuralgia after treatment, requiring medication. Sixty-three percent of patients maintained serviceable hearing (pure tone average <50 dB; speech recognition score >50%) at last follow-up. These patients also completed questionnaires evaluating dizziness, tinnitus, headache, and general quality of life. The GKS group had no decline on any component of the health status questionnaire compared with before treatment. Moreover, there was no difference in tinnitus or headache at any time comparing microsurgery with GKS. The final tumor control rate at last follow-up was 96%. As of 2013, more than 700 patients have been treated with GKS for VS in our practice.

A comprehensive review of the literature, including both retrospective and prospective studies,[6–15] shows similar favorable results, with the incidence of a new facial nerve weakness ranging from 0.0% to 6.1%, hearing preservation rates of 43% to 74%, and radiosurgical failure rates ranging from 1.4% to 10.8%. Hasegawa and colleagues[14] reviewed their long-term outcomes (median follow-up, 12.5 years) in 440 patients who underwent GKS for VS with a median tumor margin dose of 12.8 Gy. The actuarial progression-free survival at 5 and greater than or equal to 10 years was 93% and 92%, respectively. No patient developed treatment failure more than 10 years after treatment. Of 287 patients treated at a dose of less than or equal to 13 Gy, 3 (1%) developed facial palsy, and 3 (1%) developed facial numbness. Collectively, based on our own experience and that in the literature, we counsel patients with sporadic VS that single-fraction GKS with a tumor margin dose of 12 to 13 Gy has a 92% to 95% chance of long-term tumor control with a very low risk of adverse facial or trigeminal nerve outcome.

Hearing Preservation

In 2010 Yang and colleagues[11] published a systematic review of the literature evaluating hearing preservation following GKS for VS. Among 4234 patients with a mean follow-up of 44.4 months (median 35 months) the overall percentage of patients with serviceable hearing was 51%. Similarly, Hasegawa and colleagues[13] reported hearing outcomes at a median follow-up of 38 months among 117 patients treated with a mean marginal dose of 12.4 Gy. These investigators found an actuarial hearing preservation rate of 55% at 3 years and 34% at 8 years.

Long-term audiometric follow-up is particularly relevant for these patients because hearing deterioration seems to follow a protracted course compared with other cranial nerve morbidity.[13,15] Nevertheless, studies following GKS and reporting median audiometric follow-up data beyond 5 years are rare, and this is further complicated by discrepancies in how hearing outcome is reported. We recently reviewed our long-term outcome in 44 patients with serviceable pretreatment hearing (defined as American Association of Otolaryngology – Head and Neck Surgery class A or B).[16] All patients underwent GKS for sporadic VS treated with 12 or 13 Gy to the 50% isodose line, and the mean duration of audiometric follow-up was 9.3 years. We controlled for age-related decline over this long follow-up by using the nontumor contralateral ear as a control. The Kaplan-Meier estimated rates of serviceable hearing at 1, 3, 5, 7, and 10 years following GKS were 80%, 55%, 48%, 38%, and 23%, respectively.

This observation is important because data from studies with inadequate follow-up may lead to the inaccurate assumption that hearing loss following GKS for VS is exclusively an early phenomenon that levels off after the first several years. Our observations show that hearing loss following GKS continues to decline even 10 years after treatment.

Several factors, such as young patient age, low radiation dose to the cochlea, and small tumor size, have been favorably associated with hearing outcome following GKS. However, the only factor that has been consistently shown to be critical in durable hearing preservation after GKS is the presence of excellent pretreatment hearing.[15]

Dose to the Cochlea in Hearing Preservation

Recently, significant attention has been paid to cochlear radiation dose as a critical and potentially modifiable prognostic factor for hearing preservation following GKS. Several reports have identified thresholds ranging from 3.0 Gy to 5.3 Gy, beyond which there is a correlation with loss of serviceable hearing.[3,12,13,17–24] However, from a practical standpoint, if the tumor extends out to the fundus of the internal auditory canal, it is often impossible to completely cover the tumor with the prescribed radiation dose while maintaining the cochlear dose below these thresholds. We recently evaluated the relevance of cochlear radiation dose in 59 patients undergoing GKS with serviceable pretreatment hearing using more accurate CT-based volumetric cochlear dose calculations.[3] Following multivariate analysis, again, only excellent pretreatment hearing was most predictive of preserved serviceable hearing despite the cochlear dose. Although reducing the radiation dose to the cochlea may play some role in improving hearing outcomes after GKS, this may necessitate reducing the margin dose or intentionally undertreating the lateral portion of the tumor. However, these strategies may run the risk of compromising long-term tumor control.

Radiographic Follow-up after Gamma Knife Stereotactic Radiosurgery

A positive treatment response after GKS typically shows clearing of the central enhancement of the target (**Fig. 2**). This clearing can typically be seen approximately 6 months after the GKS procedure. Tumor control following GKS is defined as absence of tumor growth or a reduction in tumor volume after treatment. The imaging changes

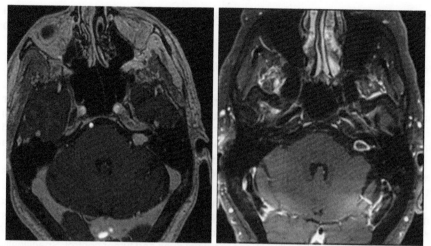

Fig. 2. Axial gadolinium-enhanced MRI at the time of VS radiosurgery (*left*) and 6 months after stereotactic radiosurgery (*right*), which shows a decrease in tumor size and enhancement. The tumor margin dose was 13 Gy.

observed after radiosurgery can be variable and must be interpreted correctly to ensure that the procedure is not prematurely deemed a failure. Tumor expansion after VS radiosurgery is common and rarely denotes a failed procedure, and most patients only require further imaging.[2,25] Approximately 5% of tumors enlarge relative to their pretreatment tumor size after radiosurgery, but do not show sequential growth on follow-up imaging.[26] As such, additional tumor treatment should be reserved only for patients who show progressive tumor enlargement on serial imaging.

Gamma Knife Stereotactic Radiosurgery for Large Vestibular Schwannomas

Typically, GKS is reserved for tumors smaller than 3 cm in linear posterior fossa diameter. Several studies have documented increased morbidity following GKS for larger tumors, but most of these tumors were treated with higher tumor margin doses (16 Gy) than is now generally used.[8,9,27–29] We recently reviewed our experience treating patients with VSs larger than 2.5 cm in posterior fossa diameter and identified 22 patients treated between 1997 and 2006. The median tumor margin dose was 12 Gy.[30] No patient had symptomatic brainstem compression at the time of GKS. The median treated tumor volume was 9.4 cm³ (range, 5.3–19.1 cm³) and the median maximum posterior fossa diameter was 2.8 cm (range, 2.5–3.8 cm). The 5-year actuarial rate of tumor control, freedom from new facial neuropathy, and preservation of functional hearing after GKS were 82%, 85%, and 28%, respectively in this subset.

The median GKS treatment volume in the 4 patients who met the criteria for GKS failure was 9.6 cm³ (range, 8.2–19.1 cm³). One death occurred during follow-up. This 59-year-old man had a rapidly enlarging tumor 7 years after GKS.[31] The patient underwent microsurgical debulking, and pathologic analysis identified the mass as a pleomorphic sarcoma; the patient died 3 months from the time of microsurgery. The other 3 patients who fulfilled the criteria for GKS failure required ventriculoperitoneal shunt placement within 1 year of surgery, and the tumor in each case subsequently failed on radiographic criteria as well. To date, just 1 lesion has required microsurgical removal, and 2 others continue to be radiographically monitored. Corticosteroid therapy for symptomatic radiation-induced changes in the brainstem and/or cerebellum was required in 3 patients (14%) for a median of 12 weeks. However, multi-variate analysis did not identify a specific feature predictive of treatment failure for these larger tumors treated with GKS.

Neurofibromatosis Type 2–associated Vestibular Schwannoma and Gamma Knife Stereotactic Radiosurgery

The natural history of neurofibromatosis type 2 (NF2)–associated VS is poorly under-stood. Previous series have reported variable outcomes, depending on the definition of tumor control and length of follow-up.[32–37] Rowe and colleagues,[36] from Sheffield, United Kingdom, evaluated 122 NF2-related VSs (96 patients) and estimated that, at 8 years after treatment, 50% of VSs lacked discernible growth. Phi and colleagues[34] reported an actuarial tumor control rate of 66% and a hearing preservation rate of 33% at 5 years.

We recently published our experience on 26 patients with 32 NF2-related VSs who underwent GKS.[32] Eighty-four percent of NF2-associated VSs showed growth arrest or tumor regression after GKS at a median follow-up of 7.6 years for the entire series. A notable association was found between marginal dose and tumor control. Specifically, the median marginal dose for tumors decreasing in size after GKS was 15.5 Gy compared with 13 Gy for tumors that enlarged after treatment, suggesting that NF2-associated VS may be best managed with higher marginal doses than those used for sporadic VS. Despite favorable tumor control, the useful hearing preservation rate was only 25% in the treated ear. These data corroborate earlier studies suggest-ing that GKS provides tumor control in approximately 80% of NF2-associated VSs at 5 years; however, hearing preservation was seen in less than 40% of treated tumors.

Risk of Malignant Transformation after Gamma Knife Stereotactic Radiosurgery for Neurofibromatosis Type 2–associated Vestibular Schwannoma

Great concern has been raised regarding the possibility of malignant tumor transfor-mation after radiation in patients with NF2 given their lack of a tumor suppressor gene. There have been 9 reported cases of malignant transformation of VS and 29 reported cases of malignant peripheral nerve sheath tumor (MPNST) after radiation therapy for VS (both radiosurgery and conventional radiotherapy).[38] Of the 29 cases of MPNST that occurred after radiation treatment, 11 of 26 patients (40.7%) in whom there was available information had neurofibromatosis (NF). An independent study in patients with NF revealed that, in a population of 1348 patients with NF2, 106 would have received radiosurgery.[39] Malignant transformation occurred in 5 of these cases, corresponding with a risk of 4717×10^{-5}; a greater risk than that found in patients who do not have NF2. However, among 14 potential cases of histologically verified intracranial malignancy arising in a stereotactically irradiated field, only 4 patients had NF2.[40] At present, although the available information suggests that there is a risk of malignant transformation caused by radiosurgery, patients should be reas-sured that the risk is very low.[38]

Cochlear Implantation after Gamma Knife Stereotactic Radiosurgery for Neurofibromatosis Type 2–associated Vestibular Schwannoma

An important and unique potential of using GKS to treat NF2-associated VSs is the ability to maintain an anatomically intact cochlear nerve, thus enabling them to become candidates for cochlear implantation.[41,42] We have taken advantage of this concept and have placed ipsilateral cochlear implants in 3 patients with NF2 after GKS for VS. The mean age of these patients was 68 years, and they had been deaf in the implanted ear for up to 10 years before cochlear implantation. All patients experienced significant restoration of hearing after cochlear implantation, achieving greater than 85% correction on hearing in noise-sensitive testing. Although microsurgery followed by auditory brainstem implantation remains our preferred method in managing VS in patients with NF2 with tumors greater than 2.5 cm, GKS followed by cochlear implantation remains an effective strategy in select patients with NF2 with smaller growing tumors.

Cystic Tumors

Cystic VS may represent a unique subtype of tumor. Although the mechanism of cyst formation is still unclear, it is postulated that recurrent microbleeding or osmosis-induced expansion of cerebrospinal fluid in trapped arachnoid may be part of the pathogenesis.[14] One important difficulty in evaluating outcomes of these tumors after GKS is trying to decide what percentage of the tumor needs to be cystic for it to be considered a truly cystic tumor. Furthermore, there is also some speculation that radiation can induce delayed cyst formation with radiation-induced repeat micro-bleeding, increased vascular permeability, or by scarring of arachnoid adhesions in irradiated tumors.[43,44] Pendl and colleagues[45] noted that 3 of 6 cystic VSs had rapid and significant expansion of the cysts that required surgery after GKS. Delsanti and colleagues[46] reported on 54 cystic VSs, of which 6.4% required additional treatment; approximately 3 times what they report for noncystic tumors. In our experience, and in the small numbers in the literature, there does not seem to be any increased cranial nerve morbidity in treating cystic VS in select patients, and tumor control seems to be favorable. Nonetheless, taking into account a potentially higher failure rate of GKS for cystic VSs, our preference is to manage predominantly cystic tumors with microsurgery.

Repeat Radiosurgery

Once a patient has failed GKS, further tumor-directed therapy is warranted. Overall, we do not favor retreating a patient with GKS after failing GKS as an initial treatment. Although our experience, and that of other surgeons, acknowledges a higher morbidity with microsurgery of VS after failed GKS,[47] that is our recommended strategy in patients who have failed primary GKS. However, there are patients who, because of significant perioperative morbidity, may be candidates for repeat GKS. To date, there are limited data on repeating GKS to the same tumor after treatment failure.[48,49] Overall, it seems that repeat GKS may be a safe and effective option in select patients for small tumors using current marginal doses (12–13 Gy).

STEREOTACTIC RADIOSURGERY FOR GLOMUS JUGULARE TUMORS

Glomus jugulare tumors (GJT) are rare neoplasms with an overall incidence of ~1 in 1.3 million people.[50,51] Nonetheless, these tumors represent the second most common tumor of the temporal bone. They are highly vascularized tumors that arise from the paraganglia of the chemoreceptor structures of the lower cranial nerves. GJTs secreting catecholamines occur in 1% to 3% of all cases. Treatment options generally include microsurgery, endovascular embolization, fractionated radiotherapy, and stereotactic radiosurgery, alone or in combination. Despite advances in all these strategies, treatment of patients with GJTs remains controversial.

Complete surgical resection is generally reserved for younger patients with large tumors causing significant mass effect. Cytoreductive resection may prove useful in those with secretory tumors with high levels of circulating catecholamines, although this remains a matter of debate. Our experience and that of other high-volume centers has shown stereotactic radiosurgery with the Gamma Knife to be highly effective with regard to low risk of cranial nerve morbidity and excellent tumor control.[52–64] Given the growing evidence showing the safety and effectiveness of GKS, many centers now support the use of radiosurgery as a primary treatment of GJT.

Dose and Tumor Control

Our technique for GKS in patients with GJTs is similar to that for VS described previously (**Fig. 3**). The expanded reach of most contemporary radiosurgical platforms (eg, the GK Perfexion) permits radiosurgical delivery to the extracranial cervical component of the tumor, at least to an inferior component of approximately the C2 level. In general, we recommend the marginal dose to be at least 15 Gy to ensure tumor control, and should not exceed 20 Gy to avoid radiation-related morbidity to the cranial nerves. In a recent multicenter study under the auspices of the North American Gamma Knife Consortium (8 Gamma Knife treatment centers), overall tumor control was achieved in 93% of 132 patients at a median follow-up of 50.5 months after GKS,[63] with a median dose to the tumor margin of 15 Gy. In patients who had upfront radiosurgery (83 patients), the actuarial tumor progression–free survival was 97% at 1 year, 89% at 3 years, and 86% at 5 years after GKS. For patients undergoing salvage radiosurgery after at least 1 resection (51 patients), the actuarial tumor progression–free survival was 98% at 1 year, 93% at 3 years, and 90% at 5 years after GKS. However, there was no difference in terms of progression-free survival between patients undergoing upfront versus salvage radiosurgery. A meta-analysis by Ivan and colleagues[57] found the pooled tumor control rate after GKS to be 95%. Similarly, a recent series of 75 patients with GJT treated with GKS, with a mean follow-up of 86.4 months, showed a volumetric tumor control rate of 94.8%.[64]

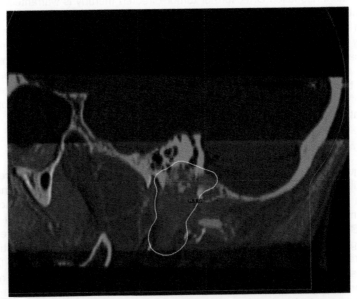

Fig. 3. Sagittal fused gadolinium-enhanced SPGR MRI and stereotactic CT showing the dose plan for a right-sided GJT. The tumor margin dose was 15.5 Gy (*yellow outline*). Note the relationship of the cochlea (*purple outline*) to the 50% isodose line.

Tinnitus and Lower Cranial Nerve Morbidity

In the multicenter study by Sheehan and colleagues,[63] 53 patients (40%) reported tinnitus at the time of GKS. After radiosurgery, tinnitus improved in 26 (49%) of these patients. New tinnitus developed in only 1 patient (0.8%) after radiosurgery. Similarly, Gandia-Gonzalez and colleagues[64] reported complete resolution of tinnitus in 54% of their patients following GKS.

Review of the literature shows the incidence of a new lower cranial nerve deficit following GKS for GJT to range from 9% to 16%.[57,63] In the meta-analysis by Ivan and colleagues,[57] the morbidities of surgery and GKS were compared. In that study, 869 patients were separated into 4 groups according to the treatment they had received: subtotal resection, gross total resection, subtotal resection combined with GKS, or GKS alone. Patients undergoing GKS alone experienced the lowest rates of recurrence of these 4 groups. In addition, the incidence of lower cranial nerve deficits was higher in gross total resection than in those who underwent GKS alone. Among 132 patients in the multicenter study by Sheehan and colleagues,[63] the overall incidence of a new cranial nerve deficit or worsening of a preexisting cranial nerve deficit was 15%. In addition, the development of a new or worsening cranial nerve deficit after GKS was a good predictor of delayed tumor growth after treatment. Hence, careful and long-term clinical and radiographic follow-up is imperative after GKS in these patients. Overall, GKS can be used as a primary treatment of GJT or in patients with recurrent disease. GKS affords a high rate of tumor control and a low risk of neurologic morbidity for patients with these tumors.

REFERENCES

1. Leksell L. The stereotaxic method and radiosurgery of the brain. Acta Chir Scand 1951;102:316–9.
2. Pollock BE. Management of vestibular schwannomas that enlarge after stereotactic radiosurgery: treatment recommendations based on a 15 year experience. Neurosurgery 2006;58:241–8 [discussion: 241–8].
3. Jacob JT, Carlson ML, Schiefer TK, et al. Significance of cochlear dose in the radiosurgical treatment of vestibular schwannoma: controversies and unanswered questions. Neurosurgery 2014;74:466–74 [discussion: 474].
4. Link MJ, Driscoll CL, Foote RL, et al. Radiation therapy and radiosurgery for vestibular schwannomas: indications, techniques, and results. Otolaryngol Clin North Am 2012;45:353–66, viii–ix.
5. Pollock BE, Driscoll CL, Foote RL, et al. Patient outcomes after vestibular schwannoma management: a prospective comparison of microsurgical resection and stereotactic radiosurgery. Neurosurgery 2006;59:77–85 [discussion: 77–85].
6. Friedman RA, Kesser B, Brackmann DE, et al. Long-term hearing preservation after middle fossa removal of vestibular schwannoma. Otolaryngol Head Neck Surg 2003;129:660–5.
7. Chopra R, Kondziolka D, Niranjan A, et al. Long-term follow-up of acoustic schwannoma radiosurgery with marginal tumor doses of 12 to 13 Gy. Int J Radiat Oncol Biol Phys 2007;68:845–51.
8. Hasegawa T, Fujitani S, Katsumata S, et al. Stereotactic radiosurgery for vestibular schwannomas: analysis of 317 patients followed more than 5 years. Neurosurgery 2005;57:257–65 [discussion: 257–65].
9. Pollock BE, Lunsford LD, Kondziolka D, et al. Outcome analysis of acoustic neuroma management: a comparison of microsurgery and stereotactic radiosurgery. Neurosurgery 1995;36:215–24 [discussion: 224–9].

10. Regis J, Pellet W, Delsanti C, et al. Functional outcome after gamma knife surgery or microsurgery for vestibular schwannomas. J Neurosurg 2002;97:1091–100.
11. Yang I, Sughrue ME, Han SJ, et al. A comprehensive analysis of hearing preservation after radiosurgery for vestibular schwannoma. J Neurosurg 2010;112:851–9.
12. Kano H, Kondziolka D, Khan A, et al. Predictors of hearing preservation after stereotactic radiosurgery for acoustic neuroma. J Neurosurg 2009;111:863–73.
13. Hasegawa T, Kida Y, Kato T, et al. Factors associated with hearing preservation after gamma knife surgery for vestibular schwannomas in patients who retain serviceable hearing. J Neurosurg 2011;115:1078–86.
14. Hasegawa T, Kida Y, Kato T, et al. Long-term safety and efficacy of stereotactic radiosurgery for vestibular schwannomas: evaluation of 440 patients more than 10 years after treatment with gamma knife surgery. J Neurosurg 2013;118:557–65.
15. Carlson ML, Jacob JT, Pollock BE, et al. Long-term hearing outcomes following stereotactic radiosurgery for vestibular schwannoma: patterns of hearing loss and variables influencing audiometric decline. J Neurosurg 2013;118:579–87.
16. Committee on Hearing and Equilibrium guidelines for the evaluation of hearing preservation in acoustic neuroma (vestibular schwannoma). American Academy of Otolaryngology-Head and Neck Surgery Foundation, INC. Otolaryngol Head Neck Surg 1995;113:179–80.
17. Link MJ, Pollock BE. Chasing the Holy Grail of vestibular schwannoma management. World Neurosurg 2013;80(3–4):276–8.
18. Brown M, Ruckenstein M, Bigelow D, et al. Predictors of hearing loss after gamma knife radiosurgery for vestibular schwannomas: age, cochlear dose, and tumor coverage. Neurosurgery 2011;69:605–13 [discussion: 613–4].
19. Lasak JM, Klish D, Kryzer TC, et al. Gamma knife radiosurgery for vestibular schwannoma: early hearing outcomes and evaluation of the cochlear dose. Otol Neurotol 2008;29:1179–86.
20. Massager N, Nissim O, Delbrouck C, et al. Irradiation of cochlear structures during vestibular schwannoma radiosurgery and associated hearing outcome. J Neurosurg 2007;107:733–9.
21. Timmer FC, Hanssens PE, van Haren AE, et al. Gamma knife radiosurgery for vestibular schwannomas: results of hearing preservation in relation to the cochlear radiation dose. Laryngoscope 2009;119:1076–81.
22. Wackym PA, Runge-Samuelson CL, Nash JJ, et al. Gamma knife surgery of vestibular schwannomas: volumetric dosimetry correlations to hearing loss suggest stria vascularis devascularization as the mechanism of early hearing loss. Otol Neurotol 2010;31:1480–7.
23. Baschnagel AM, Chen PY, Bojrab D, et al. Hearing preservation in patients with vestibular schwannoma treated with gamma knife surgery. J Neurosurg 2013;118:571–8.
24. Yomo ST, Carron R, Porcheron D, et al. A quantitative comparison of radiosurgical treatment parameters in vestibular schwannomas: the Leksell Gamma Knife Perfexion versus Model 4C. Acta Neurochir (Wien) 2010;152:47–55.
25. Nagano O, Higuchi Y, Serizawa T, et al. Transient expansion of vestibular schwannoma following stereotactic radiosurgery. J Neurosurg 2008;109:811–6.
26. Delsanti C, Roche PH, Thomassin JM, et al. Morphological changes of vestibular schwannomas after radiosurgical treatment: pitfalls and diagnosis of failure. Prog Neurol Surg 2008;21:93–7.

27. Chihara Y, Ito K, Sugasawa K, et al. Neurological complications after acoustic neurinoma radiosurgery: revised risk factors based on long-term follow-up. Acta Otolaryngol Suppl 2007;(559):65–70.
28. Foote RL, Coffey RJ, Swanson JW, et al. Stereotactic radiosurgery using the gamma knife for acoustic neuromas. Int J Radiat Oncol Biol Phys 1995;32:1153–60.
29. Kondziolka D, Lunsford LD, McLaughlin MR, et al. Long-term outcomes after radiosurgery for acoustic neuromas. N Engl J Med 1998;339:1426–33.
30. Milligan BD, Pollock BE, Foote RL, et al. Long-term tumor control and cranial nerve outcomes following gamma knife surgery for larger-volume vestibular schwannomas. J Neurosurg 2012;116:598–604.
31. Schmitt WR, Carlson ML, Giannini C, et al. Radiation-induced sarcoma in a large vestibular schwannoma following stereotactic radiosurgery: case report. Neurosurgery 2011;68:E840–6 [discussion: E846].
32. Mallory GW, Pollock BE, Foote RL, et al. Stereotactic radiosurgery for neurofibromatosis 2-associated vestibular schwannomas: toward dose optimization for tumor control and functional outcomes. Neurosurgery 2014;74:292–300 [discussion: 300–1].
33. Sharma MS, Singh R, Kale SS, et al. Tumor control and hearing preservation after gamma knife radiosurgery for vestibular schwannomas in neurofibromatosis type 2. J Neurooncol 2010;98:265–70.
34. Phi JH, Kim DG, Chung HT, et al. Radiosurgical treatment of vestibular schwannomas in patients with neurofibromatosis type 2: tumor control and hearing preservation. Cancer 2009;115:390–8.
35. Subach BR, Kondziolka D, Lunsford LD, et al. Stereotactic radiosurgery in the management of acoustic neuromas associated with neurofibromatosis type 2. J Neurosurg 1999;90:815–22.
36. Rowe JG, Radatz MW, Walton L, et al. Clinical experience with gamma knife stereotactic radiosurgery in the management of vestibular schwannomas secondary to type 2 neurofibromatosis. J Neurol Neurosurg Psychiatry 2003;74:1288–93.
37. Mathieu D, Kondziolka D, Flickinger JC, et al. Stereotactic radiosurgery for vestibular schwannomas in patients with neurofibromatosis type 2: an analysis of tumor control, complications, and hearing preservation rates. Neurosurgery 2007;60:460–8 [discussion: 468–70].
38. Seferis C, Torrens M, Paraskevopoulou C, et al. Malignant transformation in vestibular schwannoma: report of a single case, literature search, and debate. J Neurosurg 2014;121(Suppl 2):160–6.
39. Baser ME, Evans DG, Jackler RK, et al. Neurofibromatosis 2, radiosurgery and malignant nervous system tumours. Br J Cancer 2000;82:998.
40. Carlson ML, Babovic-Vuksanovic D, Messiaen L, et al. Radiation-induced rhabdomyosarcoma of the brainstem in a patient with neurofibromatosis type 2. J Neurosurg 2010;112:81–7.
41. Lustig LR, Yeagle J, Driscoll CL, et al. Cochlear implantation in patients with neurofibromatosis type 2 and bilateral vestibular schwannoma. Otol Neurotol 2006;27:512–8.
42. Carlson ML, Breen JT, Driscoll CL, et al. Cochlear implantation in patients with neurofibromatosis type 2: variables affecting auditory performance. Otol Neurotol 2012;33:853–62.
43. Park CK, Kim DC, Park SH, et al. Microhemorrhage, a possible mechanism for cyst formation in vestibular schwannomas. J Neurosurg 2006;105:576–80.

44. Pollock BE, Brown RD Jr. Management of cysts arising after radiosurgery to treat intracranial arteriovenous malformations. Neurosurgery 2001;49:259–64 [discussion: 264–5].

45. Pendl G, Ganz JC, Kitz K, et al. Acoustic neurinomas with macrocysts treated with gamma knife radiosurgery. Stereotact Funct Neurosurg 1996;66(Suppl 1): 103–11.

46. Delsanti C, Regis J. Cystic vestibular schwannomas. Neurochirurgie 2004;50: 401–6 [in French].

47. Slattery WH 3rd. Microsurgery after radiosurgery or radiotherapy for vestibular schwannomas. Otolaryngol Clin North Am 2009;42:707–15.

48. Dewan S, Noren G. Retreatment of vestibular schwannomas with gamma knife surgery. J Neurosurg 2008;109(Suppl):144–8.

49. Yomo S, Arkha Y, Delsanti C, et al. Repeat gamma knife surgery for regrowth of vestibular schwannomas. Neurosurgery 2009;64:48–54 [discussion: 54–5].

50. Heth J. The basic science of glomus jugulare tumors. Neurosurg Focus 2004;17: E2.

51. Guss ZD, Batra S, Li G, et al. Radiosurgery for glomus jugulare: history and recent progress. Neurosurg Focus 2009;27:E5.

52. Eustacchio S, Trummer M, Unger F, et al. The role of gamma knife radiosurgery in the management of glomus jugular tumours. Acta Neurochir Suppl 2002;84:91–7.

53. Feigl GC, Horstmann GA. Intracranial glomus jugulare tumors: volume reduction with gamma knife surgery. J Neurosurg 2006;105(Suppl):161–7.

54. Ganz JC, Abdelkarim K. Glomus jugulare tumours: certain clinical and radiological aspects observed following gamma knife radiosurgery. Acta Neurochir (Wien) 2009;151:423–6.

55. Genc A, Bicer A, Abacioglu U, et al. Gamma knife radiosurgery for the treatment of glomus jugulare tumors. J Neurooncol 2010;97:101–8.

56. Gerosa M, Visca A, Rizzo P, et al. Glomus jugulare tumors: the option of gamma knife radiosurgery. Neurosurgery 2006;59:561–9 [discussion: 561–9].

57. Ivan ME, Sughrue ME, Clark AJ, et al. A meta-analysis of tumor control rates and treatment-related morbidity for patients with glomus jugulare tumors. J Neurosurg 2011;114:1299–305.

58. Liscak R, Vladyka V, Wowra B, et al. Gamma knife radiosurgery of the glomus jugulare tumour - early multicentre experience. Acta Neurochir (Wien) 1999;141: 1141–6.

59. Miller JP, Semaan M, Einstein D, et al. Staged gamma knife radiosurgery after tailored surgical resection: a novel treatment paradigm for glomus jugulare tumors. Stereotact Funct Neurosurg 2009;87:31–6.

60. Miller JP, Semaan MT, Maciunas RJ, et al. Radiosurgery for glomus jugulare tumors. Otolaryngol Clin North Am 2009;42:689–706.

61. Sharma MS, Gupta A, Kale SS, et al. Gamma knife radiosurgery for glomus jugulare tumors: therapeutic advantages of minimalism in the skull base. Neurol India 2008;56:57–61.

62. Varma A, Nathoo N, Neyman G, et al. Gamma knife radiosurgery for glomus jugulare tumors: volumetric analysis in 17 patients. Neurosurgery 2006;59:1030–6 [discussion: 1036].

63. Sheehan JP, Tanaka S, Link MJ, et al. Gamma knife surgery for the management of glomus tumors: a multicenter study. J Neurosurg 2012;117:246–54.

64. Gandia-Gonzalez ML, Kusak ME, Moreno NM, et al. Jugulotympanic paragangliomas treated with gamma knife radiosurgery: a single-center review of 58 cases. J Neurosurg 2014;121:1158–65.

Index

Note: Page numbers of article titles are in **boldface** type.

Otolaryngol Clin N Am 48 (2015) 527–532
http://dx.doi.org/10.1016/S0030-6665(15)00044-4
0030-6665/15/$ – see front matter © 2015 Elsevier Inc. All rights reserved.

oto.theclinics.com

Moving?

Make sure your subscription moves with you!

To notify us of your new address, find your **Clinics Account Number** (located on your mailing label above your name), and contact customer service at:

Email: journalscustomerservice-usa@elsevier.com

800-654-2452 (subscribers in the U.S. & Canada)
314-447-8871 (subscribers outside of the U.S. & Canada)

Fax number: 314-447-8029

Elsevier Health Sciences Division
Subscription Customer Service
3251 Riverport Lane
Maryland Heights, MO 63043

*To ensure uninterrupted delivery of your subscription, please notify us at least 4 weeks in advance of move.

Printed and bound by CPI Group (UK) Ltd, Croydon, CR0 4YY

22/10/2024

01777783-0003